Neuroplasticity, Memory, and Sense of Self

Neuroplasticity, Memory, and Sense of Self

An Epistemological Approach

Mirko Di Bernardo

Translated by Peter Waymel

The Davies Group, Publishers

Aurora, Colorado

Library of Congress Cataloging-in-Publication Data

Di Bernardo, Mirko.
Neuroplasticity, memory and sense of self : an epistemological approach / Mirko Di Bernardo.
pages cm
Includes bibliographical references and index.
ISBN 978-1-934542-41-5 (alk. paper)
1. Neuroplasticity. 2. Cognitive neuroscience. I. Title.
QP363.3.D53 2013
612.8'233--dc23
2013037964

Translated from the Italian by Peter Waymel

0123456789

To my parents and Arianna, to whom I owe all that I am,
to Francesca with immense love,
to Aurelio Simone with affection, esteem and deep gratitude

Contents

Great is the power of memory, a frightening thing, Oh my God, a deep and boundless multiplicity; and this thing is the mind, and I am this thing.

— St. Augustine

If we do not understand how the mind is based on matter, scientific knowledge and the knowledge of ourselves remain separated by an abyss. Building a bridge over this abyss is not impossible. However, biology and psychology teach us that it is made of many parts. How do we know? How do we feel? A philosophical statement, however deep, cannot contain the answer, which instead must arise from an understanding of how biological systems and biological relations have evolved in the physical world.

— Gerald M. Edelman

Omne verum, a quocumque dicatur, a Spiritu Sancto est.

— St. Thomas Aquinas

Preface

As the brain-changes are continuous,
so do all these consciousnesses
melt into each other like dissolving views.
Properly they are but one protracted consciousness,
one unbroken stream
— William James, The Principles of Psychology

The development of non-invasive monitoring technologies for neuroscience has led in just a few years to the detailed understanding of a large number of brain processes revealing their integrated and multi-layered complexity. The interdisciplinary debate characterizing the cognitive science domains, which seemed originally to be guided (1978, first issue of *Cognitive Science*) by computer science and by the mathematical models of its "armed wing," artificial intelligence, today sees a leadership on the part of neuroscience that has marked a definitive and irreversible shift from positions centered on the concept of algorithms to other positions oriented towards the systemic nature of collective behavior in dynamic networks. The physics of emergence (the undersigned is a theoretical physicist) has played a decisive role in showing the inadequacy of mechanistic reductionism that was heavily present in the symbolic models of early cognitivism, drawing attention to the subtle problems posed by open systems and system-environment relations (Licata, 2008; for a general review cf., for example, Licata, Sakaji, 2008).

Contrary to what one might expect, the rise of experimental knowledge did not lead to a renewal of the current paradigms in cognitive science, which still seems to linger amid the old physicalist and computationalist schemes, whose reductionist flavour is only thinly disguised by an appeal to their greater "biological plausibility." In other words, it seems that the cognitive complexity is still a "complication" waiting for new theoretical scenarios and perspectives of meaning able to shed new light on the enormous amount of experimental evidences.

It is not a coincidence if we still argue about "brain mechanisms," thus revealing a privileged attention to a search for "laws of thought" while actually ignoring the implications of procedural and contextual aspects of cognitive activity. Such aspects are closely linked to the question of *embodiment* and we can therefore say that giving up the vision of mind as a "control centre of representations" requires developing sufficiently structured theories capable of meeting the "ecological" challenge of the mind-in-the world and transforming the Fodor's provocative remark into a stimulating *modus tollens*: "If that is what nonrepresentational, embodied, ecological cognitive science is all about, I'll stick with computationalism. Maybe I'll become a pastry chef instead" (J. Fodor, cited in Chemero, 2009).

The essential point is to understand that an embodied approach to cognition must be able to put at its core a theory of emergence similar to the one physics developed over the past decades. A theory of this kind regards the organism-environment system as a single entity in "structural coupling" from the beginning (Maturana, Varela, 1992), taking into account the organism's actions on the environment and the environment's actions on the organism, and framing cognition as a *historical process* that emerges from the collective behavior of "neuronal mechanisms" immersed in the stream of experience. A truly complex system is a system where the dynamics are triggered by the boundary conditions, and not fixed once and for all by some sort of original wiring. The many measures of complexity proposed in literature integrate those of information and entropy, and aim to characterize how a group of interconnected subsystems modify themselves under suitable conditions and constraints, showing forms of emergence (phase transitions, levels of auto-hetero-organization, functional consistency).

It is clear that such a philosophy does not aim at detailed predictions or a "final" classification of cognitive structures (similar to a theory of everything in physics), but tends rather to understand the conditions and modalities in which a cognitive activity actually takes place. The need for a systemic approach was perceived in the study of vision ever since the times of Gestalt psychology, which had put the emphasis on the global features of the process. This kind of approach answers the question posed later by Gibson (Gibson, 1986): *The rules that govern behavior are not like laws enforced by an authority or decisions made by a commander: behavior is regular without being regulated. The question is how this can be.* Similar problems, unassailable by the old symbolic approaches, can be found in the study of memory that, far from being a data storage mechanism, has proved to be a fine reconstructive process in which the "fluid" stratification of previous experiences of the cognitive agent and its adaptation needs are tied in a metastable state. The emergentist approach to cognition seems thus to be the only one able to fuse structural aspects and functional dynamics into a single vision , so including in a natural way one of the greatest achievements of the encounter between biomathematics and neuroscience, the stochastic neuroplasticity of the *noisy brain* (Deco et al., 2009; Deco, Rolls, 2010).

Another question on which classical cognitivism seems to be stranded is that of information. If the new cognitive science has to be based on what we know of the brain, then it is appropriate to ask whether the Shannon-Turing computational model is the most suitable one to describe the characteristics of the informational flow in cognitive processes. Being by now dismissed von Neumann's digital neuron and its many descendants, there exist manifold evidences that biological activity, at any scale, involves both discrete and continuous aspects (Van Rullen, Koch, 2003; Huys et al. .2008), and is characterized by processes of *semantic* appropriation of information based on the organism's *history* and ruled by the emergence of new codes (Cariani, 2011). In a syntactic theory of information there is no room for uncertainty, but the brain works at its best in such condition. (Doya et al., 2011). In other words, in order to study cognitive emergence it is necessary to develop an approach to information which can include the *meaning* and *purpose* of behavioral scenarios. This has spurred a systematic and structured retrieval of analog computation within a vast area that goes by the name of *natural computation* (Rozenberg et al., 2012). Here we limit simply to mention "field computation" or "morphic computation," which uses the deformation of a suitable parametric space as an "indicator" of the informational flow between system and environment. So we go at the core of the term 'information' ("to give form"), in accordance with R. Milner: *Computing is transforming our environment*. The goal, in line with *Intelligence without Representation* by R. Brooks, and L. Steels, is that of a *geometry of biological information* that can take into account also semantic aspects such as emerging forms (Resconi, 2013).

The questions of meaning naturally lead us to the hard problem of consciousness. Here too one has the impression that the hardest aspects arise more from classical cognitivism's expulsion of radical subjectivity and *qualia* than from the intrinsic inapproachability of the topic. Even quantum physics has been invoked (with some *ad hoc* corollaries and a few forced assumptions) to explain consciousness, but it is precisely the evidence of neuroscience that shows us, once again, the need for a vision of emergent complex integration (Scott, 1995). If anything, there is a persistent epistemological confusion between "theories of consciousness" (in the third person) and experience of consciousness (in the first person) that continues to cause rivers of ink to be spilt, a frantic activity that could be conveyed towards more fruitful directions if only scientists wished to truly follow the magisterial lecture on neuro-phenomenology of the essentially unheard Varela (Gallagher, Zahavi, 2008).

Finally, since who writes a preface can allow himself a greater degree of freedom than the author can do with his broad and precise work, I would like to close my notes with a (technical) observation and a guess on the future of cognitive science, with the hope that the author will appreciate them. If the mind is not in Putnam 's vat, then we must follow what embodiment, intelligence without representation and neuro-plasticity reveal to us. There is no "mind" without the subtle play of orientating in the world that is given by radical subjectivity and the selective complexity of emotions, volitions, beliefs. Even the new generations of scholars of robotics—who seem the ones most distant from the topic of consciousness—have realized this, so that today there is an entire research field, that of artificial consciousness, where the possibility of making artificial systems more versatile is studied, trying to induce them to a different and "plural" relationship with experience (Haikonen, 2007). It is thus not difficult to imagine that the consciousness William James posed as the central element of his program of scientific psychology, having exited cognitivism's metaphorical door, might today recover its centrality, thanks to neuroscience, as the organizing principle of experience, the cognitive compass of the encounter between the mind and the world.

The author of this book, Mirko Di Bernardo, is a new generation philosopher of biology. He knows that epistemology is not a moment *external* to scientific research but an activity of analysis and critique that is an integral part of the process of scientific production. His text is actually extremely detailed about the most advanced aspects of the brain sciences, and unites with crystalline clarity the theoretical and experimental facets of neuroplasticity with their philosophical implications. Mirko is a biographer, pupil and friend of Stuart Kauffman, and in this book he not only seems to answer some of the questions raised by Stu regarding cognitive science (Kauffman, 2009), but shows the same ability to ask questions and to trigger problems, an attribute which is, or should be, the peculiar feature of a scientist, when he recalls that he is also a natural philosopher.

Ignazio Licata
Professor of Theoretical Physics
ISEM, Inst. for Scientific Methodology,
Palermo, Italy.

Acknowledgments

This book would not have been possible without an abundance of help. I am first indebted to Ignazio Licata, who accepted to write the preface; its enlightening reflections enhance this book considerably. I am also extremely grateful to Giuseppe Tanzella-Nitti and Philip Larrey for the great generosity and deep humanity with which they have helped me publish this book, by suggesting the publishing house, and I offer my deepest thanks to the publisher, The Davies Group, Publishers, for choosing to value the work of a young scholar. The book owes its existence first of all to their invaluable encouragement.

I have been helped enormously also by conversations with A. Carsetti, S. Kauffman, F. Jimenez Rios, E. Baccarini, M.G. Marciani, E. Pessa, N. Baccin, M. Durst, D. Palomba, F. Tempia, M. Buzzoni, A. Strumia, C. Cirotto, M. Buiatti, G. Basti, F. Santoianni, A. Montanari, L. Floridi and M. Oliva.

A special thanks goes to Peter Waymel for the competence and professionalism with which he translated this volume. And I am once again indebted to Francesca Lattuneddu for her help at the editorial level. Moreover I would particularly like to thank James K. Davies for the editorial comments and suggestions that have contributed to the quality of the presentation of the book.

A heartfelt thanks goes to the Centre for the Interdisciplinary Documenting of Science and Faith of the Pontifical University of the Holy Cross, and in particular my friends at the Advanced School for Interdisciplinary Research (ADSIR) with whom I had the opportunity to discuss and share many inspirations arising from this work.

I also thank G. Boffi, director of the SEFIR research area of the Ecclesia Mater Institute of Rome for allowing me, by organizing various conferences, to delve into many themes treated in this book.

My deepest thanks go also to my students of the "Tor Vergata" University of Rome for their stimulus, their interest and for their patience.

I will always be grateful to Franco Miano and Stefano Semplici, my teachers. I have learned much from them, and continue to do so every day. Without their friendly support, I would never have found the courage to embark on the difficult path of research that has led to this book.

Chapter 1

Neurophysiological Aspects of Consciousness

1.1 Premise

At the beginning of the twenty-first century cognitive science branched out, separating into various types of cognitive sciences that integrated with other, neighboring scientific approaches. But more significantly, the field as a whole showed the signs of a profound paradigm shift. The theoretical model of reference during the cognitive sciences' initial phases of development, since the 1950s, is the computationalist model based on a comparison, considered accurate by some, inaccurate by others, of the human cognitive apparatus to a digital computer. This schema has for more than twenty years now been the object of a growing dissatisfaction within the field of cognitive science theory. Today, in fact, given the crisis regarding the theoretical guidelines laid down by the computer metaphor, the orientation emerging in the cognitive sciences does not merely recognize the highly distributed and connective nature of all neural processes, but goes so far as to explicitly reject the idea of a cognitive apparatus that functions according to an input-output schema. That is, it refuses the idea of the mind as a processor of pre-existing, pre-selected information (within a space of predefined alternatives) as well as the conception of knowledge as something that proceeds by way of symbolic calculations, producing copies of the outside world. In other words, the emerging paradigm, which some scholars have called "embodied cognition" (Lakoff, Johnson, 1999; Lakoff, Nuñez 2001; Damasio, 1999; Edelman, 2004), distances itself from abstract knowledge, knowledge separated from the emotional sphere and independent from intentionality and agency. Today, therefore, the cognitive sciences and, more generally, the sciences of mind can no longer simply produce an abstract model to apply and vary according to individual biological situations; rather, they must identify a field of processes and highly contextual emergences, which it is the job of research and often of the various disciplines to place in relation in such a way as to cause useful questions to arise.

Traces of this change in perspective are very evident today in pedagogy's new exploratory dimension, in virtue of the field's gradual hybridization with scientific approaches and methodologies proper to the life sciences, the philosophy of mind, and, in particular, neuroscience. Over the past twenty years, in fact, research in educology has been gradually moving towards recovering the biological dimension of the teaching-memorizing-learning relationship. This epigenetic dimension (and, more generally, the interpretative considerations of pedagogy-neuroscience) has been understood as constitutive of individual uniqueness and, therefore, has proven to be an ineluctable step in the processes of planning, managing and developing educational dynamics. When the notion of a possible link between pedagogy and neuroscience was conceived, it carried with it some anti-reductionist reservations, such as, for example, its distancing of itself from functionalist positions, which hold that the functions of the mind can do without their biological substrate and be implemented in any computing device (Frauenfelder, 2001; Frauenfelder, Santoianni, Striano, 2004).

We can also view as anti-reductionist reservations the recognition of the correlational character mediating the complex mind-brain link, going beyond the simplistic interpretations alleging a mere coincidence between brain activations and mental events and beyond, moreover, every vision of mind that does not take into account a plurality of perspectives and that is not multi-dimensional.[1] Given this situation, the current research into cognitive function, has since the end of the last century in the broadest sense been moving away from the computational matrix which had originally generated such studies, drawing ever closer to an interpretation of the mind as embodied, situated and distributed (Varela, Thompson, Rosch, 1991; Varela, 1999). A mind that can no longer be studied separately, in itself, but in an increasingly integrated way, by considering the dynamic unity of its parts correlating it to the brain, to the body, and making it, together with them, an organism, just as we ought to consider "organismic" its synergistic and interactive situation with the environment, which includes it, contains it and, at the same time, specifies and distinguishes it (Sabatano, 2004). Consequently, the idea that a cognitive agent is something centralized and unified has been replaced by the concept of a "disunified" self. The modules, in fact, are incomprehensible to cognitive experience and lack access to consciousness and introspection (Santoianni, 1998). From here it emerges that the cognitive self is not represented by a totality, but by a series of emerging units from this disunified network (Siegel, 2001; Zeki, 2011). In light of this, therefore, the cognitive process now arises as an emergence of form, not a shaping of form. It is morphogenesis in act that is no longer reducible to genetic programming. It is unpredictable, not algorithmic. It is complexification and sophistication. In short, it is a process, not a simple result (Santoianni 1994, Frauenfelder, 2001). A formative hypothesis must therefore head in the direction of a globality in which the relational channel becomes a participant in strategic operations, and in operations of organizing and selecting through the information mass (Bruner, 1986, 1993). In this sense, the scenario of educational research is enriched with new lines of research that can offer tools for elaborating hypotheses in this direction, but that, precisely for this reason, can and should make use of the most recent contributions of cognitive science, neurobiology and philosophy (Santoianni, 1998, 2003).

Beyond this theoretical horizon of reference, the scientific starting point of the research presented in this book, though revisited within an epistemological framework and particularly from within J. Hintikka's revisitation (1970) of the concept of semantic information, originally outlined by Carnap and Bar Hillel in 1952 (a revisitation that developed, in the sixties and seventies, a theory of depth information that significantly broadened the horizon of Carnap's original assumptions, to the point of addressing the same problem of finding a possible determination of the content of semantic information at the level of polyadic structures). Almost simultaneously, in the seventies and eighties, algorithmic information theory, following in the wake of Kolmogorov's (1965) and Chaitin's (1974) original studies, was outlining its theoretical connotations with particular regard to the issues of incompleteness and incompressibility, coming finally to attentively re-examine Gödel's (1972) original findings. These theoretical developments were soon grafted onto the issues of cognitivism and connectionism: the result was the real possibility of a new approach to the problem of delineating the path of the construction of knowledge, an approach capable of taking into account, in a significant manner, that particular interweaving of incompressibility, on the one hand, and meaning on the other, that constitutes the connective tissue of the human mind (Carsetti, 2004). This approach resulted, in the Nineties, in the birth of a specific version of complexity theory, able to take into consideration the problem of the very constitution, throughout the course of natural and cultural evolution, of the mental operations that characterize objective knowledge. The theoretical frameworks mentioned above have led in recent years to the progressive opening of new and fruitful horizons for research, also for what concerns the realm of the mind sciences (Freeman, 2000a, 2008; Freeman, Vitiello, 2009). Specifically, this book addresses the theme of memory from a threefold perspective.

First, at the neurophysiological level, this study focuses on identifying the structure and functions of memory in the transition from the vegetative to the minimally conscious state, thus offering new and important insights regarding the study of alterations of consciousness and the new frontiers of rehabilitation (Kandel, Pittenger, 2003; Kim *et al.*, 2003; Owen *et al.*, 2009).

Second, at the epistemological level, the results of neuro-scientific research are contextualized and re-interpreted in a philosophical key, looking, moreover, to focus on the mysterious relationship that exists, at the level of the meaning-oriented construction of higher-order conceptual spaces, between semantic memory, cognition and intentionality (Freeman, 1994, 1997, 2000b, Searle 2004, 2008; Carsetti, 2009b). With regard to the possibility of creating such a model of the process of rational perception, the scientific community finds itself today before a new frontier, one closely linked to the emergence of a conceptual revolution at the level of the analysis of that particular entanglement of complexity, information, causality, meaning, emergence, teleology and intentionality that characterizes the unraveling of the "natural forms" of human cognition (Carsetti, 2009a; Petitot, 2013). A revolution based on an examination of the new measures of information related to the "semantic code" of the mind, devised in recent years through analysis done by several research groups in Europe and the United States. The exploration of some of the specific regions of this particular frontier constitutes one of the objectives of this present work.

Third, at the phenomenological and neuropedagogical level, in order to furnish an effective definition of educational processes and their related practices, the investigation of memory cannot fail to consider the importance of the qualitatively distinct and multi-factorial nature of the mnestic system (Sabatano, 2004, 2005; Strollo, 2008). This type of survey would allow us to acquire the data needed to define individualized learning paths within which to create *different settings* for strengthening and balancing peoples' mnestic qualities. Finally, in the concluding section we will try to develop, at the epistemological and neuroscientific level, a comparison between the methods of developing the mnestic abilities just mentioned and the phenomenological category of empathy (Gallese, 1996, 2008; Rizzolatti *et al.* 2006; Boella, 2005).

In these circumstances, therefore, we can rightly infer that the theme of memory is by definition interdisciplinary, and lies generally at the intersection of several studies of a psycho-pedagogical, bioneuroscientific, phenomenological and epistemological nature, also becoming one of the privileged objects of study within the broader paradigm of complexity theory (Kauffman, 1993; Maturana, Varela, 1980; Siegel, 1999; Freeman, 2000a). Over the last few years, this theory has aroused the attention of the international scientific community since it can be regarded as the epistemological base of departure for a new approach to the mind/body problem, an approach that is able to hold together—while maintaining distinct—the various levels of reference, the holism of the sciences of the spirit, and the methodological reductionism of the natural sciences. Through the use of this particular epistemological approach, therefore, this volume focuses on cutting edge issues relating to the close relationship between cognition and life, issues such as: synaptic plasticity (the basis of memory and cognition), the relationship, at the level of the higher cognitive activities proper to human beings, between perception, thought and sense of self on the one hand, and the nature of intentionality on the other, the difference between consciousness and self-consciousness, and the genesis of meaning in the context of the deep processes of self-organization.

Finally, in regard to memory, it seems possible to link the idea of a "transversality" of levels of thought (related among themselves and which can be related to the parallel activation of neural networks and their expression in synchronized mental operations) to research on the plurality of cognitive and functional levels and, in this sense, it is possible to combine the consideration of the multifactorial, quantitatively and qualitatively distinct nature of learning with the corresponding multifactorial, synergistic and integrated nature of memory (Pessa, Vitiello 1999; Vitiello Pessa, 2003; Kandel, 2009). Memory, in this perspective, is understood as having a distributed functioning, composed of different processing methods and pertaining to different natural domains, among which pride of place goes to particular modulating systems that cooperate in larger brain processing areas such as the limbic system and the neocortex. The limbic system and neocortex have been considered the depositary brain areas of emotional processes and cognitive processes, respectively, areas entrusted with different levels of processing. These processing levels, however, albeit distinguishable, seem to be deeply interconnected; and it is precisely in the areas of possible linkage between the limbic system and the neocortex that neuroscience research has located nervous nuclei involved in learning and memory processes (Owen *et al.,* 2005; Posner *et al.,* 2009; Damasio, 2010). The presence of subcortical areas common to both the limbic system and the neocortex has shown experimentally the inseparability of the emotional from the cognitive, and vice versa (Jaynes, 2000; Vecchiato *et al.*, 2009). As a result, writes C. Sabatano (2005), their mutual collaborative interaction has brought about (in the various interpretations of the mind and its relationship with the brain) both a "cognitivization of the concept of emotion," and an "emotionalization of thought." The emotional, therefore, becomes cognitive, is represented by this dimension and, at the same time, contains the cognitive within it and can regulate its expression, in the sense that the emotional can exert a hierarchical control of a metareflexive nature over the cognitive (Beauregard *et al.*, 1998).

1.2 Memory and the neurosciences

The ability to memorize information is necessary for learning, adaptation and thus for the survival of all living organisms, from bacteria to human beings. Without memory an organism could react only to current stimuli, being unable to learn from past experiences or make predictions about the consequences of its own behavior. This function, in the course of evolution, has developed a great deal of flexibility and complexity, forming ever closer and more and articulate ties with other mental functions such as learning, thinking, the emotions and motivations. On the last rungs on the evolutionary ladder, memory becomes more and more the psychic structure that organizes behavior in a perspective that is both temporal (establishing links between past and present and anticipating the future) and causal (establishing deterministic or probabilistic links between two related events), going so far as to involve the very organism itself and allowing, moreover, it to construct its own identity thus as a particular self-consciousness.

Therefore, in the human being, learning, memory and consciousness are inextricably linked. Most of our notions about the world around us are not present in the brain from birth, but are acquired through experience and retained thanks to memory. In this sense, we are what we are thanks in large part to what we make experience through learning. Memory allows us, moreover, to receive an education and it constitutes a powerful driving force for the growth of society's consciousness. The human being has the unique ability to communicate to others what he has learned and, in doing so, is able to create a cultural heritage that can be passed down from one generation to another. In the last three decades there has been a real revolution in what we know about memory and the processes that occur in the brain when we learn and remember. In the first three chapters of this book, in addition to tracing the exciting origins of this revolution, we will show the main findings concerning mnemonic activities and the activities of nerve cells and brain systems. The smallest unit of memory is the mnestic trace, a modification created by a previous event that influences a subsequent event. The experimental study of memory, begun in the late nineteenth century with the experiments of Ebbinghaus, thus concerns the understanding of the specific mechanisms that characterize each phase of memory. Typically, three phases are distinguished: encoding or learning; storage; remembering, retrieval, reactivation and actualization. During the first phase, that of encoding or learning, the individual memorizes certain responses aroused by the demands of the context in which he finds himself, resulting in the formation and organization of mnestic traces. The second phase, storage, consists in the latent retention of what has been memorized and extends for a variable period of time during which certain chemical and physical changes occur. In the last phase, remembering, retrieval, reactivation and actualization, the previously acquired responses are retrieved and may result in observable mnemonic behavior: one can see what has been retained and how (Beauregard *et al.*, 1998). Mnemonic pathways can be divided into three broad categories: remembrance, recognition, and relearning. The first category, remembrance, includes the reproduction of responses learned in a previous situation, and narration, by which the subject becomes aware of a past experience. In the second category, recognition, the subject identifies a past situation in which he responded in a certain way or identifies a previously memorized object present in his current perceptual field. The third category, relearning, allows one to infer the presence of processes of retention, and therefore the existence of a mnestic trace, through economy of exercise: the time and effort necessary to repeat the learning are generally less than the first time the thing was learned (Craik, Tulving, 1975).

A subject's access to these categories of observable mnemonic pathways naturally depends on several factors, including the duration and quality of the subject's learning, the more or less conscious strategies adopted during retention, the subject's motivation and individual aptitudes; factors that jointly contribute to the strength of the mnestic trace. A person's mnestic performance will therefore differ according to the method used to test their degree of retention (Siegel, 1999). With recognition, the mind compares a current process with a trace from a previous event (greater retention value). During reconstruction, the recovery of the mnestic trace is facilitated by the mind's presenting some element of the material that initially caused the trace (Kandel, 1979b, 2001, 2007). During retrieval, one recalls a memory through a special internal tension that seeks to bring to the level of consciousness a trace that may be deeper or shallower (lower retention value).

What has been said so far clearly shows how, in the neurosciences, the study of memory today is based on two different approaches. The first refers to the biological study of how nerve cells communicate with each other. The key discovery here, which we shall examine later in detail, was that the communication between nerve cells is not fixed, but can be modulated by activity and experience. Therefore, an experience can leave a memory in the brain; it does so by using the nerve cells as basic memory storage devices (Kandel, 1979a, 1983a, 1983b, 2005, 2009, 2012). The second approach, however, concerns the study of brain systems and cognitive abilities. The most important finding in this regard is that there is not a single type of memory, but that there are different types that follow different logics and use different brain circuits (Tulving, 1972; Collins, Loftus, 1975; Fodor, 1975, Squire, 2004, 2007). The first two chapters of this work attempt to combine these two historically distinct approaches to propose, in agreement with Squire and Kandel (2009), a new synthesis: a molecular biology of memory, which highlights the interaction between the molecular biology of neural communication and the cognitive neuroscience of memory. Some of the processes to be described are derived from studies on memory and on learning in the neural circuits of simple invertebrates, while others come from studies of more complex nervous systems, including that of the human brain.

Among the recent technological advances that have enabled us to deepen our knowledge of memory and consciousness is the ability to monitor the human brain while a person is learning and remembering. In this way, we are able to link elements involved in cognitive functioning to specific brain areas. This task is carried out thanks to the development of powerful methods for studying the internal representation of cognitive processes. Specifically, as we shall see in the next paragraph, scientists are now able to record the activity of brain cells in wakeful animals intent on exhibiting particular behaviors, and to obtain images of the human brain of individuals engaged in specific cognitive activities, by means of the positron emission tomography (PET) and functional magnetic resonance imaging (fMRI). Together, these developments have allowed us to study the processes taking place in the brain when people receive sensory stimuli, perform motor activity, learn and remember. A now classic example of such research, at the clinical and neurophysiological level, is that of recent studies on human beings carried out by Laureys and Owen (Laureys, 2004, 2007; Owen, 2013, 2008; Monti *et al.*, 2010) with regard to the transition from the vegetative state to the minimally conscious state. These developments show how the biology of memory can be studied today not only at the level of cellular and molecular mechanisms of the storage of information, but also and primarily at the level of brain structure, brain circuits and behavior, i.e., the neural systems involved in memory.[2]

1.3 Clinical aspects of consciousness

The nature of consciousness has been the subject of great philosophical interest at least since the days of classical Greece. Only in the last century, however, have assumptions regarding the basis of consciousness been influenced by our knowledge of the functional mechanisms of the central nervous system. The properties of consciousness are however very difficult to explain from a scientific point of view. Clinicians, therefore, rely on a pragmatic conception based on the individual's ability to respond appropriately to environmental stimuli. Numerous clinical observations have shown that the ability to properly orient oneself towards stimuli depends on the totality of activities in the two cerebral hemispheres. When certain regions of the cerebral cortex are injured, the ability to process certain types of information is lost, causing the subject in this way to lack awareness of some aspects of his or her environment. According to this view, therefore, in order for generalized disorders of consciousness to occur, there must be a functional alteration of both hemispheres of the brain.

The alteration of consciousness, therefore, is one of the most difficult and dramatic clinical problems. In ancient times, the Greeks knew that a normal state of consciousness requires an intact brain, and altered consciousness means brain damage. When faced with a disturbance of consciousness, the limited time available for a physician to act and the many possible causes of brain injury represent a challenge for him, and at the same frighten both him and the patient's family members. Progress in the medical-scientific field in the last fifty years has enabled the human being to survive renal, cardiac and respiratory problems which until then had always left no way out. This has made it possible to keep patients alive who otherwise would inevitably have faced death. But increased chances of survival brought with them new problems, creating clinical situations previously unknown. It is thus that in these last few years, we have witnessed the appearance of low response states and consciousness disorders such as the Vegetative State (VS) and the Minimally Conscious State (MSC). These are clinical conditions in which vital functions are maintained thanks to the support of artificial treatments, while the cognitive abilities are partly, and often irremediably, compromised. To define the relationship between the two nosographic categories—VS and MSC—it is necessary first to examine how the neurosciences define consciousness: it is "the state of full awareness of oneself and one's relationship with the surrounding environment" (Posner *et al.*, 2007). Most of the time, determining a patient's state of consciousness is a challenging task for a doctor. At the clinical level, the assessment of the state of consciousness is done based on the answers the patient manages to give the doctor. It can happen that the patient is conscious but unresponsive, as occurs in locked-in syndrome or in those cases where for psychological reasons the subject refuses to respond.

There are two main components to consciousness. The first regards the content of consciousness, and involves the set of functions of the cerebral cortex, including the cognitive and affective functions. The corresponding anatomical bases of these functions are unique networks of cortical neurons; it is thus possible for a lesion to a strategic point to create an interruption responsible for a partial loss of consciousness while the subject still manages to perceive other stimuli. In such cases (partial disturbances of consciousness), the clinician must accurately identify to which class of stimuli the cognitive or behavioural impairment refers (Marciani, Placidi, 2009). The second component is the level of consciousness, or the level of behavioral responsiveness, which is closely linked to the state of wakefulness: stem structures (diencephalon, midbrain, pons—ascending reticular substance). It is clear that cognitive functions (content of consciousness) are not possible without an appropriate level of consciousness (state of wakefulness). While a full state of consciousness is associated with the waking state, the sleep-coma binomial has always raised many questions especially from a neurophysiopathological point of view (Marciani, Placidi, 2009).

Sleep, a biological rhythm essential for survival, is a recurring form—physiological, not pathological—of reduction of consciousness. A key difference between sleep and a coma is that the former is a cyclical event, and is reversible, since a sufficiently intense stimulus is capable of bringing the individual back to a waking state. In an altered state of consciousness, depending on the state's severity, the stimulus may be totally ineffective or can result in an awakening of short duration which ceases when the stimulation itself ends (Posner *et al.*, 2007).

1.4 The vegetative state

The classic definition of coma, stated by F. Plum and J. B. Posner (2007), is the following: "a state of unarousable unresponsiveness in which the subject lies with their eyes closed." There is therefore no evidence of any psychologically understandable response to external stimuli or internal needs. In general, a coma, which rarely persists longer than four weeks, is described as a pathological condition characterized by a reduction, to the point of abolition, of the state of consciousness and responsiveness to external stimuli, with (sometimes marked) alterations of vegetative functions (such as breathing and cardiovascular activity). Current data given by the scientific community show that the longer the duration of the loss of consciousness, the less likely the recovery of functional autonomy (except for post-traumatic comas). However, the development of the artificial respirator, refined by Bjorn Ibsen in Denmark, modified the previous system of mechanical ventilation in order to offer an important support to the cardio-circulatory activity, giving many patients a chance to live through a coma from a brain injury they previously would not have survived. This intensive care technology has led to redefining death based on neurological criteria (for example, brain death) and is mainly responsible for an increased incidence of patients awakening from a situation of acute coma, though showing no signs of voluntary interaction with their environment. A few days or weeks after the severe brain injury, patients begin to open their eyes, breathe without help and make spontaneous movements or stimulus-induced reflexes. This clinical syndrome was initially called apallic syndrome or waking coma; later in 1972 it was called *Wakefulness Without Awareness* (WWA) and Persistent Vegetative State (PVS) (Calvet, Coll, 1959; Laureys *et al.*, 2010). The term "*Unresponsive Wakefulness Syndrome*" (UWS) has recently been proposed (Laureys *et al.*, 2010). Clinical practice shows the complexity involved in recognizing signs of conscious perception of the environment and of the self in patients recovering from a coma. This difficulty, confirmed by frequent misdiagnosis of *locked-in syndrome*, derives, as we have just mentioned, from the fact that an objective assessment of residual brain function is extremely difficult in patients with severe brain damage due to either a partial or total absence of their motor responses (Marciani *et al.*, 1996; Marciani, 2011).

In addition to this clinical evidence, we must keep in mind two important aspects, namely, that consciousness is not an *all-or-nothing* type phenomenon (but, rather, should be conceived as a continuum between different stages) and also that there is a theoretical limit to the certainty of our diagnosis, since we can merely infer the presence or absence of a conscious experience in another person (Tong, Thakor, 2009). From the clinical standpoint, the patient in VS never shows behavior that testifies to the awareness of himself (and of the surrounding environment), active exploration, communication, expression or comprehension of language or purposeful movements oriented towards external or internal stimuli. These patients are not, however, completely unreactive: they can move their trunk or limbs, they may occasionally smile, and, on even more rare occasions, moan. Yet we are unable to identify in these components any voluntary responses, the evidence of self-awareness; in short, these gestures display no recognizable elements of communication (Posner *et al,* 2009). The key element in diagnosing a patient as being in VS is thus their *unresponsiveness.* Yet performing a diagnosis based on an *indirect* criterion of consciousness is limited by the fact that consciousness increasingly appears to be a *continuum* that is difficult to reduce to a series of clearly-defined states, delineated on the basis of purely behavioral elements (Marciani, Placidi, 2009).

The name VS refers to the preservation of nervous vegetative functioning, which means these patients also preserve intact their sleep-wake cycles, breathing, digestion and thermoregulation (Gosseries *et al.*, 2011). The term *persistent* (PVS) was added to indicate that this condition has persisted beyond an arbitrary period of one month from the traumatic or non-traumatic brain injury. Despite there being no sure criteria for establishing when VS becomes permanent, and its being difficult to diagnose (because we are dealing with patients with heavily damaged cerebral hemispheres, while their brainstem is relatively well-preserved), the guidelines for determining a prognosis when a patient is in VS have made considerable progress in recent years as a result of large-scale retrospective studies done by the *Multisociety Task Force on PVS*[3] whose report suggests that a VS that continues for 12 months subsequent to TBI, or for 3 months subsequent to anoxic damage, should be considered permanent. However, this view is not shared by the entire scientific community.

It is important to note that a small number of patients may recover from VS past the above-mentioned time limits, though these late instances of recovery of consciousness are always accompanied by severe disability. Clinical analysis, diagnostic imaging (EEG, evoked potentials) and morphological imaging are insufficient for reliably predicting the prognosis of a patient in VS. Scientists' motivation for using functional imaging on patients in VS twofold: first, because patients in a vegetative state represent an important clinical problem in terms of diagnosis, prognosis, treatment and daily management, and second, because this technique offers a lesional approach to the study of human consciousness, making a valuable contribution to the research effort in order to identify the neural correlates of consciousness. Indeed, these patients represent clear cases of an abolition of responsiveness with wakefulness intact, contrary to what is observed in comatose patients (Posner *et al.*, 2007). As we shall see in the next paragraphs, the results of these studies, comparative in nature, in these last few years have seemed to confirm the hypothesis that consciousness depends on the ability of different brain areas to influence each other dynamically (Laureys, 2005, 2007; Laureys, Schiff, 2012; Owen, 2013). In other words, consciousness would seem to depend on the unfolding of a continuous and bidirectional dialogue between the primary and the associative cortical areas. Specifically, the development of techniques able to "hear" inner dialogue directly in the brain has represented a significant step forward for the diagnosis and understanding of disorders of consciousness in patients with severe brain injury, by highlighting the existence of individuals who, despite suffering from severe brain injury, are still able to express, albeit sporadically, the presence of some form of consciousness (Boly *et al.*, 2011).

1.5 The minimally conscious state

In 1996, the *Aspen Neurobehavioral Workgroup*, taking into consideration the large number of diagnosis errors concerning VS,[4] proposed that a new diagnostic category be introduced: the Minimally Conscious State, or MCS. This new category would be diagnosed on the evidence of purposeful behavioral signs that would allow one to infer the presence in the patient of a minimal degree of awareness of their environment (Andrews *et al.*, 1996). The MCS[5] is generally associated with a series of characteristic clinical features including the presence of sleep-wake cycles and the partial presence of awareness. It is important to note, however, that consciousness in these patients 'fluctuates,' so it is possible for there to be long periods of non-conscious wakefulness. In fact, patients in MCS can exhibit a variety of behaviors that, though fragmented, repeat and are protracted over time, highlighting the presence of intentionality and, therefore, are distinguishable to the clinical eye from simple automatic or reflexive replies (Posner *et al.*, 2007).

Spontaneous eye opening, without the recovery of consciousness or of voluntary motor behavior, indicates the transition from coma to VS. Instead, the patient's transition from VS to MCS is marked by manifesting voluntary behaviour[6] which the patient is able, moreover, to repeat. Such behavior includes staring at visual stimuli and/or tracking the same with their gaze, executing simple commands, making yes/no verbal or gestural responses, uttering intelligible words or making purposeful motor activity in relation to environmental stimuli. As related by Posner and other scholars, moreover, the emergence from MCS towards a condition of severe disability is indicated by the return to functional interactive communication and/or by the ability to use objects in a functional way (at least two different objects) (Posner *et al.*, 2009). The transition from a severe degree of disability to a condition of moderate disability is marked by a return to a personal autonomy sufficient for independent living. The return to work or school indicates a desirable level of recovery has been achieved. For some patients in MCS, their cognitive functioning remains in good condition, though it fluctuates over time. For precisely this reason, some scholars have proposed other definitions of MCS, such as: *minimally responsive state* and *state of minimal awareness* (Bernat, 2002). A state of minimal responsiveness, measured at the patient's bedside, can, as mentioned before, conceal discrete cognitive functioning, even up to situations of normal cognition, such as that observed in *locked-in syndrome.*[7]

Another important aspect is the evaluation of late recoveries from MCS. Often the public confuses comas and VS, particularly with regard to both diagnosis and prognosis. From the data obtained from retrospective studies by the Multisociety Task Force, it has emerged that the majority of cases of recovery have been in fact late *transitions* not from a coma or VS, but from MCS. At present there is insufficient data to establish guidelines regarding the duration of MCS (Giacino *et al.*, 2002). What does seem confirmed by the results of recent research and comparative studies on patients in MSC and VS, instead, is the need of the international scientific community to identify, through the use of increasingly sophisticated technologies, an objective measure of the neural correlates of consciousness (Tononi, 2004, 2012). Such a measure would increase diagnostic precision enormously, especially for those patients who, despite being conscious, are unable to move because of more or less extensive injuries to their motor systems. It is in this direction, for example, that the current collaboration between Massimini's group at the University of Milan and the *Coma Science Group* at Liège University Laureys is working; the groups have developed a project that shows how by measuring communication between brain areas we can distinguish patients in VS from patients who have recovered a minimum level of consciousness (MCS) (Raina *et al.*, 2012). It is important to note that this measure can be obtained at the patient's bedside and requires neither full functioning of the patient's sensory pathways or motor skills nor their ability to understand or carry out commands. The results of the work may have significant consequences in the clinical field since the distinction between VS and MCS patients is so difficult that it leads to diagnostic error in a full 40% of cases.[8] We'll see shortly how at the basis of these important studies, which today more than ever are seriously laying the groundwork to try to begin to understand in an increasingly complex and profound way how the brain is able to generate consciousness, there is the use of specific technologies able to expand drastically the depth of clinical observation, resulting also in a real paradigm shift in the diagnosis and prognosis of disorders of consciousness (Cruse, Owen, 2010).

1.6 Functional diagnosis of states of consciousness

Scientists involved in brain function imaging,[9] particularly using fMRI[10] and PET, have shown a growing interest in the diagnosis and prognosis of disturbances of consciousness such as VS and MCS (Laureys *et al.*, 1999, 2000; Laureys, 2004, 2005, 2007; Owen *et al.*, 2006, 2007). In the absence of a clear understanding of the neural correlates of consciousness, even a "near normal" activation in response to passive stimulation (visual, auditory, somatosensory) can be difficult to interpret in terms of unequivocal proof of consciousness. One can only conclude that a specific area of the brain is somehow still able to activate and process sensory stimuli. This is of great interest not only from a neurophysiopathological and clinical point of view for the purposes of diagnostic and prognostic evaluation of VS and SMC, but also because of the bioethical and epistemological implications of these two states. One of the main objectives of this review, therefore, is to probe the alleged "pillars of Hercules" of the contemporary mind sciences: namely, the frontier regarding the close relationship between cognition and life and, at the level of higher cognitive activity, human perception, thought and sense of self, the nature of intentionality and the difference between consciousness and self-consciousness.

In this sense, the experimental studies that I will refer to in this volume constitute a veritable scientific heritage whose philosophical implications have not yet been fully explored. For example, the studies on both pathological and pharmacologically-induced[11] comas have revealed a common factor underlying both types of coma: damage to the activity of a diffused cortical network that includes associative parietal cortices but not the "lowest level" sensory cortices (Coleman *et al.*, 2009). At any rate, one important finding, as Dehane, Tononi, Noirhomme and other scholars all have demonstrated independently, is the evidence that a "decrease in regional activation" seems insufficient to explain loss of consciousness, which requires a further "functional disconnection" within that network and in its relationships with the thalamus. Therefore, conscious awareness depends in a selective manner on the functional integrity of the thalamocortical and cortico-cortical frontoparietal connectivity within the networks and between the cerebral networks themselves (Tononi *et al.*, 2004; Tononi, 2012; Dehaene *et al.*, 2006; Noirhomme, *et al.*, 2010).

In the last few years the study of brain connectivity has allowed scientists to begin to shed light on some of the mechanisms that underlie disorders of consciousness: wakefulness and awareness. To understand connectivity, it is necessary to think of brain activity as an activity based on the processing of information in a modular and distributed manner. Brain functions can thus be analyzed through the identification of neuronal *pools* and the analysis of their relations. In such a view, the brain appears as a synergistic set of multiple interacting subsystems, each dedicated to a particular function (Marciani, 2011). The consequence of this assumption is that differences in brain activations during different experimental conditions arise in general from different neuronal dynamics, both in terms of their spatial cortical localization and of the variation of the functional links between the cortical areas themselves. In other words, cortical regions activated in similar ways may produce different behavioral and/or cognitive responses on the basis of differences in their functional links alone (Freeman, 2004, 2006, 2007).

As we have intimated in the preceding paragraphs, over the last decade the development of non-invasive methods for mapping brain activity based on hemodynamic measurements (functional Magnetic Resonance Imaging, fMRI) or electromagnetic measurements (HR-EEG, at high resolution; magneto electroencephalography, MEG) has allowed us to deepen our knowledge of brain areas activated during motor or cognitive tasks in humans. However, an important question that still remains open today is that of the mode of communication between the various brain regions. In this regard, the concept of cortical connectivity plays a central role in neuroscience, as it represents a possible means of understanding the coordinated functioning of the cortical regions, beyond their mere activation (Marciani, Placidi, 2009). Various definitions of connectivity have been proposed: one of them defines functional connectivity as the measure of the temporal correlation between brain activities in distinct areas of the brain, without, however, inferring any causality between these activities. Several algorithms have been proposed for evaluating functional connectivity, starting from high resolution EEG data, and followed by data from PETs and fMRIs (Cincotti *et al.*, 2003, 2007, 2008). The methods for evaluating cortical connectivity, validated through simulation, use mathematical models able to support the evidence that *wakefulness* is not correlated to the activity of a single brain region but to the thalamocortical network within the fronto-parietal network (Di *et al.*, 2008). Therefore, the integrated study of functional connectivity utilizing functional imaging data (electrophysiological, hemodynamic, metabolic) is currently a very helpful diagnostic tool to understand the residual functional capacity in the brain in the process of perception and integration, essential in distinguishing between PVS and MCS in diagnosis.[12] Recently, on the basis of new evidence, the suggestion has been made to create a further diagnostic category, between VS and MCS, called *non-behavioral MCS* (Schiff, 2006). The problem of accurately diagnosing VS is therefore still characterized by controversial elements and, regardless of the discussion about the possible persistence of "hidden consciousness," in some of these patients, all the evidence of recent years seems to indicate that the conditions of cortical activity in patients with a clinical diagnosis of PVS are anything but invariably absent or minimal (Owen *et al.*, 2006, 2007; Owen, 2008, 2013). In any case, one must take into consideration that at least one subset of VS patients, as some very recent studies seem to suggest, and which we will examine later on, retains a level of cortical connectivity bringing them closer to the minimally consciousness state, and that allows them to process some affective and/or cognitive elements of environmental stimuli. Taken together, however, the clinical neurological examinations and assessments of the structural integrity of the brain provide only a limited picture of the neurophysiological mechanisms of the coma, the vegetative state and the minimally conscious state. This is due to the fact that the functional changes in the populations of neurons distributed throughout the cerebral cortex, the basal ganglia and the thalamus, which are the cause of these conditions, often cannot be adequately evaluated by such methods. Nevertheless, neuroimaging techniques that can directly assess functional changes inside these brain networks, are giving rise to significant advances able to definitively improve diagnostic accuracy and our understanding of the pathophysiology of severe brain damage. The ability to identify the physiological mechanisms underlying the different functional outcomes in the context of the category of severe disability, is leading to a better understanding of the necessary and sufficient neurological results for the recovery of consciousness, and is allowing us to distinguish the different levels of cognitive ability. For example, the imaging techniques (fMRI and PET) presently being employed by different groups of researchers (Laureys-Liegi and Owen-MRC Cambridge) in evaluating patients in PVS have helped deepen our knowledge, at the neurophysiopathological level, of part of the *brain circuitry.*

In the last decade, in fact, studies done with these techniques, have allowed scientists to measure objectively the brain's *reactivity* to external stimuli in patients both in PVS and in SMC. The results have shown three modes of response in these patients:[13] a) absence of cortical activation; b) an activation typical of *low-levels* of the primary sensory cortices; c) an atypical activation that tends to spread to the *higher-level* associative cortices (Di et al., 2008). However, the passive stimulation paradigms used in the past have not allowed us to make assertions about the presence or absence of consciousness. Paradigms have recently been proposed that use *mental images* evoked by external stimuli (visual or auditory) with emotional value, to identify signs of consciousness in non-communicative patients in VS or MCS (Bekinschtein *et al.*, 2011). In the article entitled "Residual auditory function in persistent vegetative state: a combined PET and fMRI study," Owen and colleagues (2005) developed an imaging procedure for assessing voluntary responses in patients in VS and MCS that overcomes the ambiguity of previous methods. Applying this new procedure, these researchers were able to determine, beyond any possibility of error, that a patient in VS for five months after severe brain trauma was able to execute the command to imagine different visual scenes. The commands were linked with the activation of appropriate areas of the cerebral cortex, despite the absence of an external motor response. At the time of the examination, the patient showed evidence of a short fixation of his gaze, a possible sign of a transition in progress to MCS. Another patient, eleven months after brain injury, was able to perform visual tracking in a mirror, another transitional sign, but showed no signs of manipulating objects or executing commands. For this specific patient the images showed a preservation of cognitive function that the clinical examination had failed to reveal and indicated a cognitive level at least compatible with MCS.

In continuity with the results mentioned above, more experimental evidence also seems to have come from the amazing results achieved recently by Rosanova, Tononi, Laureys and Massimini who have developed a new technique that would cause research to take a huge step forward, as it enhances the ability to measure the neural correlates of consciousness. It is a technique based on the combination of Transcranial Magnetic Stimulation (TMS) and the electroencephalogram (EEG) applied to severely brain damaged patients who showed an evolution from a coma to other clinical states (Rosanova *et al.* 2012; Massimini *et al.*, 2012; Tononi, Massimini, 2013). The TMS/EEG allows one to measure directly and noninvasively the internal communication in the brain, a condition that according to theoretical neuroscience is necessary for the emergence of consciousness.

Previous studies have shown that the approach based on TMS/EEG allows one to distinguish states in which consciousness is present (alert wakefulness, dreaming) from states in which consciousness is reduced or absent (sleep, anesthesia) (Boly *et al.* 2011). In VS patients, who in terms of their behavior appear awake, having their eyes open, but are unable to respond to external stimuli, TMS/EEG shows a lack of communication between cortical areas, as observed in sleep or anesthesia; on the contrary, in MCS patients, who show minimal signs of consciousness, TMS has found that communication between cortical areas is preserved and effective, regardless of the patient's ability to communicate with the external environment. The results of this work, therefore, suggest that by "questioning" the brain directly (using TMS) to gauge its capacity for internal dialogue (using EEG) one can effectively monitor the neural correlates of the recovery of consciousness for patients with severely cerebral injury and who are unable to communicate.

In such circumstances, therefore, just as the concept of brain death has clarified for us the concept of death, so the concept of MCS is forcing us to reconsider the notion of consciousness more precisely, which today from a neuro-physiological viewpoint is defined simply as "the knowledge that an individual has of himself, his emotional life and his environment" (Posner *et al.*, 2007). This definition has been adopted for purely clinical purposes. However, from the philosophical point of view, the problem of consciousness and our understanding of it go far beyond the level of neuro-pathophysiology. Indeed, in these last few years the new functional imaging techniques for the minimally conscious state are offering important insights into the primary modulation of the semantic code of the human mind, the origin of cognition and the complex relationship between language, meaning, memory, learning and intentionality (Carsetti, 2004). It is here, as we shall see later, that the current results of neuro-physiological and neuro-psychological research on the state of consciousness (Fernández-Espejo *et al.*, 2010) and on the relationship between memory, identity and knowledge (Siegel, 1999, Freeman, 2000a; Freeman, Quian Quiroga, 2013) can be revisited, contextualized and interpreted in the light of those new categories offered by other fields of study such as, for example, the theory of self-organization and intentional complexity theory. Studies also in the context of *symbolic dynamics* promise a useful new perspective from which to interpret neuro-physiological and neuro-psychological research; in these last few years work in this field has played an important role in the ongoing efforts aimed at delineating a first reconstruction, in simulation, of those processes of continuous emergence of new structures of meaning that characterise the subsequent articulation of the procedures of human reasoning and of cognitive activity in general (Carsetti, 2013).

The surprising results of the aforementioned experimental studies performed using fMRI or TMS/EEG on patients in VS and MSC, as well as the recent and extraordinary discovery by Naci and Owen (2013) concerning the ability to dialogue using functional magnetic resonance imaging even with patients who have been clinically diagnosed as VS and who instead may prove to be conscious and able to send information to the outside world by communicating correct answers to binary (yes or no) questions,[14] leads us to rethink the relationship between cognition, consciousness, self-awareness, memory and intentionality. This discovery leads us to distinguish the "self" from self-consciousness and unconscious memory from declarative memory, and supports the idea that a physical system is conscious to the extent that it is able to "integrate biological information" (understood as form + intentionality). That is, the substratum of consciousness must be a system composed of many functionally different elements which are, however, closely linked together to form an indivisible entity endowed with unity, wholeness and purpose. This is anything but trivial: it is a delicate balance between diversity and unity that seems to evoke some ancient philosophical concepts, such as *adaequatio,* assimilation and organicity. Naturally, there are many different ideas about the neural substrates of consciousness, but basically there are those who say that consciousness depends on the activation of a specific brain area (or mechanism) and those who say that what counts is a widespread activation of a large part of the brain.

The thesis I will attempt to present in the following pages seeks to combine both aspects (specialization and integration) through the use of the key concept of intentionality, i.e. the process of continuous creation of meanings with which the individual adapts to the world thanks to the occurrence of cerebral processes which each time are unique and unrepeatable. In order, therefore, not to offer solutions, but to present better some of the most important theoretical problems being addressed today, this review will continue by showing how, parallel to the research carried out by Laureys, Owen, Tononi and Massimini (and in accordance with their results), in recent years, in neurobiology and epistemology, a number of studies are cropping up related to intentionality and the biological capacity to know and remember. In particular, in the third chapter we will make reference to Freeman (2000a, 2000b, 2008; Freeman, Quian Quiroga, 2013) and Kauffman (2000; 2008), who will show how intentionality cannot be located only at the level of consciousness, but is also present in non-conscious, autonomous agents, coming moreover to be considered one of the key features of the bios. In the fourth chapter, then, following some reflection about the neurobiology of intersubjectivity and Siegel's theory of integration (1999), as well as studies on mirror neurons mainly carried out by Rizzolatti, Sinigaglia (2006) and Gallese (2006), we will focus our attention on the fundamental concepts of multi-systemic memory and sense of self by revisiting even some traditional philosophical approaches. With respect to the possible charting of new models with regard to the process of the construction of knowledge, I will show, finally, the most recent research results related to a new frontier, closely linked with the emergence of a real revolution in terms of conceptual analysis of that particular *entanglement* of information, meaningful complexity, memory, causality and teleology that characterizes the unfolding of the natural forms of human cognition (Carsetti, 2009b, 2010a, 2012a, 2013). In this sense, for instance, the news territories of non-standard models and non-standard analysis represent, at the moment, a fruitful prospective in order to point out some of the basic concepts concerning the articulation of an adequate intentional complexity theory.

For the moment, however, I will limit myself in the next chapter to showing how, according to Kandel's and Squire's research (2009), imaging techniques associated with recent discoveries in molecular biology have allowed us to take a real leap forward in terms of the study of the "nature" and "functions" of memory both on the molecular and the cognitive level.

Chapter 2

Molecular Mechanisms of Memory

2.1 From memory as a psychological process to the biological revolution

From Ancient Greece, the birthplace of philosophy, and, in a strict sense, of ontology as the seminal element of Western thought, it was clear that man was endowed with innate cognitive faculties, that is to say, that the means through which an individual perceives the external world and constructs notions or ideas that can be expressed and shared with others is intrinsic to that same person. So from Socrates onwards, philosophy understood as the love of knowledge has attempted to find adequate answers to fundamental questions about the mystery of man's inner life and that regarding the presence of the world. Some of these questions could be summarized as follows: how do we assimilate new information about the outside world and how is such information learned and stored in the memory? What is the ultimate nature of our knowledge? Which types of human knowledge are innate and to what point does experience condition the organization of the innate faculty concerning the reorganization of our knowledge? At the beginning, the study of memory and other processes that today we would call mental was based exclusively on non-experimental methods of a philosophical. The difficulty, however, resided in the fact that these methods did not allow researchers to identify clear, empirical facts. In the mid-nineteenth century the successes of experimental science in solving problems of a physical, chemical and biological nature began to attract scholars interested in analyzing behavior and, more generally, mental faculties. Thus, with regard to the study of consciousness, in subsequent years, the philosophical survey was gradually supplemented, to the point of being almost entirely replaced, by empirical studies of mind that gave birth to psychology as a discipline independent of and distinct from philosophy and more generally by the analytical sciences.

Experimental investigation allowed researchers to begin to shed light on the role and nature of human beings in relation to other living species and in relation to the history of the Earth. In the *Origin of Species,* in fact, Darwin argued that, like morphological characteristics, mental characteristics also demonstrated continuity in different species. He then suggested that the study of animals should also make it possible to understand our mental life (Darwin, 1902, 1958). Darwin's idea that the mental capacities of our species evolved from simpler organisms inspired the successes obtained by Ebbinghaus (1885) on human memory as well as the animal models for the study of learning developed independently by Pavlov and Thorndike. Pavlov (1927) discovered classical conditioning, while Thorndike (1911) discovered operant or instrumental conditioning. In the eyes of the scientific community, these studies soon became milestones for the scientific study of memory and learning in non-human living beings.[1] This kind of objective psychological approach to learning, based on experimental methods, gave rise to the empirical tradition called behaviorism, which has transformed the way we conduct the study of memory. Under the leadership of the American, Watson (1930), the behaviorists studied and measured the response to external stimuli (behavior) through the rigorous method proper to the natural sciences. Accordingly, they claimed, psychologists should concern themselves solely with what could be observed. The problem, however, was that the nature of individual experience and of mental events is not agreeable to these realities being analyzed scientifically in this way. Nevertheless, studies in the context of this tradition on classical conditioning and instrumental conditioning have provided much useful information: the idea of reward as a key to understanding learning, the description of how different types of reward-reinforcement influence the times of learning, the motivations linked to the ways in which animals associate stimuli.

"In their attempt to emulate the natural sciences and to study only observable stimuli and responses, the behaviorists [. . .] restricted the domain of experimental psychology to a limited set of problems, and excluded from study some of the most fascinating features of mental life, such as the cognitive processes that occur when we learn and remember." (Squire, Kandel, 2009, pp. 5–6).

An important pioneer of a cognitive approach to the study of memory was the psychologist Bartlett (1951), who showed how memory is fragile and susceptible to distortion, adding a naturalistic dimension to Ebbinghaus's rigorous control methods for studying memory (Bartlett, 1958). He suggested that evoked memories are rarely accurate. Recall does not correspond to a simple rewinding of passively deposited information waiting to be repeated, but is essentially a creative process of reconstruction, and reorganization. Thanks to Bartlett's work, many psychologists had recognized the limitations of behaviorism. It was understood that perception and memory depended not only on information contained in the surrounding environment.[2]

Shifting their attention to the study of the internal dimension proper to mental operations, cognitivists tried to follow the flow of information, from the sensory organs to its internal representation-elaboration in the brain and final use in mnemonic and motor processes. It was believed that internal representation took the form of a distinctive set of activities by specific groups of brain cells connected to each other.

Information theory and the theory of the "calculating machines"—also called "computability theory"—played an important role in the development of the fundamental concepts of cognitive psychology. They highlighted how, in addition to physical entities such as the matter or energy transmitted, a key role is played in such processes by a more abstract entity, called "information."[3] This latter reality, understood as an immaterial yet measurable physical quantity, involves the way matter and energy are distributed in space and time and, more specifically, the relationship between their actual spatial-temporal distribution and the expectations of the one who interprets this distribution as a message—hence the idea of information as a "relation of the ordering of parts that could be (ordered) differently" (Wheeler, 1990). To wit, in all communications systems used so far, energy is distributed in the form of localized packages, each of which corresponds to a "symbol." This approach allows you to represent a message through a sequence of symbols—that "codify" it—and the expectations of the recipient with the probability that he assigns to the appearance of any particular symbol (Shannon, 1948). By knowing the latter it even becomes possible to characterize quantitatively the "information" associated with each message. Naturally, this characterization is always tied to a subjective element, consisting of the particular assignment of probability made by the receiver of the message. However, it becomes 'general' when this assignment is the same for a very wide class of receivers (Shannon, 1948; Penna, Pessa, 1998).

In particular, using this type of characterization of the content of "information," a human observer is able to describe the processes of transmission and processing of signals that takes place in a digital computer as though they correspond to processes of the transmission and processing of the information of appropriate messages.[4] In agreement with Pessa and Penna (2009), the widespread diffusion has contributed to linking cognitive processes with those we describe as processes of elaborating and transmitting information in digital computers, and this outlook has been gradually established in the eyes of the scientific community as the cornerstone of cognitive psychology.

In fact, the aim of this particular field of studies consists in the identification of "programs" that underlie assimilation processes such as perception, memory and learning. In such circumstances, therefore, and with such a theoretical outlook, what emerges clearly is the deep bond that unites cognitive psychology and artificial intelligence, that is, the discipline that aims to equip computers with the processing capacities similar to those of humans, to the extent that even artificial intelligence can be conceived on the technical-engineering level of the original research program of cognitive psychology. However, while this combination led to important interdisciplinary collaborations that, before the advent of the cognitivist paradigm, were basically unthinkable, such a conceptual framework raises serious difficulties, not least of which is that of defining what can serve as symbols and symbolic messages in a processing system, such as the cognitive faculties, that is conceived as being structurally similar to a digital computer only from a logical-formal (abstract) point of view, but not from a physical one. A proposed solution to this difficulty was advanced by Fodor (1975), who hypothesized a correspondence between extended sets of possible physical events and particular, individual states of mind, which served as "representatives" of the physical events that they were associated with. Fodor called these states "representational states of mind." The central idea of Fodor's theory was that each representational state was univocally associated with a symbol, such that the cognitive processes, on his view, consisted of computational processes causing one to pass from one representational state to another and, for this reason, one could say that they are reduced to processes of symbolic processing (i.e. computation) (Penna, Pessa, 1994, 1998).[5]

Man's capacity to give meaning to things has constituted, from the dawn of civilization, one of the peculiar features that distinguish our species, inasmuch as it is able to create symbols. It is therefore no coincidence that the overwhelming majority of studies on memory have been dedicated to this, man's mysterious capacity to know through conceptualization and to transmit what he knows to others through symbolic language. For the same reasons, semantic memory has also been the subject of a vast number of studies.[6] The models of its operation are divided into two categories: network models and models based on traits. The first have a significant historical importance in the development of connectionism,[7] both because they were implemented in computers, and because they are substantially equivalent to certain neural networks. In the network models (Collins, Quillian, 1968) the structure of semantic memory is represented through a network of "nodes" and "arches." The first reflect concepts, while the latter represent the connections between concepts (Penna, Pessa, 1998). In models based on traits (Meyer, 1970) each concept is defined by a number of features, or "traits" or "attributes." Thus the representation of the concept in the memory (mnestic trace) coincides with the list of attributes or traits distinguishing it (Hintzman, 1986).

These were built to interpret data arising from a series of particular experiments, all framed within a general paradigm, which can be summarized as follows: a) presentation of an affirmative or interrogative sentence that contains a particular element and a general concept; b) measure of the reaction time employed to provide the answer.

As Pessa and Penna pointedly note, the fundamental assumption behind all network models of semantic memory is that the measured response time is directly proportional to the "distance" between the concepts in the phrases used in the experiments. Attempting to represent geometrically the concepts as points or "nodes" in a hypothetical two-dimensional space, whose relative distances are proportional to the measured reaction times. If one were to highlight the distances by drawing appropriate segments or "arches" linking the various concepts, one would have Collins and Quillian's original model from 1968 (Penna, Pessa, 1998; Pessa, Penna, 2004).

This type of representation emphasizes, first, how concepts can be defined implicitly through the network of relationships that connects them to other concepts. This suggests that knowledge can be represented by recourse to models. Moreover, it provides a way to understand how the properties of particular concepts can be inferred from those of general concepts. Of course this model provides only a static description of how knowledge is organized in memory. Yet if we focus our attention on the process of retrieving the stored information, we can endow the model with its own dynamics[8].

It is not the purpose of the present study to discuss the advantages and disadvantages of network models. What I wish to say is that such models have given birth some novel ideas that later became part of connectionism and, in some respects, of the molecular biology of cognitive activities, a new paradigm that a few years later would explode thanks to the fundamental contribution of Kandel and Squire as regards in particular the study of the molecular mechanisms of learning and memory (Kandel, 1976, 1979, 1983a; Kandel *et al.*, 2000; Squire, Kandel, 2009).

According to Penna's and Pessa's reflections, the points of this paradigm can be summarized in the following five points. First, the information stored in a system can be in "distributed" form, defined implicitly by the network of interconnections existing within a set of potentially activable units; therefore, it is not necessarily concentrated in precise locations in the memory. Second, an activation pattern of a set of units is equivalent to a representation of the (temporary) state of knowledge embedded in the system. Thirdly, every interconnection between two units must be given a "label" specifying the characteristics. Fourthly, the recall of stored information understood as the issuance of a response to a particular input is the result of a process of dynamic evolution of the network, in which the momentary activation patterns of the various units change over time. Finally, by leveraging existing interconnections, the activation spreads from one unit to another with a diffusion process similar to that of a physical signal transmission from one place to another (Penna, Pessa 1998).

In the third chapter, we will come back to deepen our study on the passage from cognitivism to connectionism, and from the latter to post-connectionist perspectives that will question, at the level of living systems, the concept of information conceived solely as a message that propagates itself on a support, as in the information theories of signals or in general in the handling of information, revisiting, moreover, ancient concepts such as, for instance, that of "actuality"—the capacity to inform through a "form." For the moment, however, it is important to note only that the semantic networks do not constitute a completely "distributed" representation of information, since each node is associated with a very precise and unique symbolic sequence, which constitutes its "label." It is possible then to assert that each node contains a concentrated symbolic representation of a particular piece of information and that the process of the spreading of the activation is equivalent to a selection process—and therefore to computation—that acts on an appropriate set of symbols. From this point of view the network models fall perfectly within the cognitivist paradigm, and are not inconsistent with Fodor's interpretation (Pessa, Penna, 2004). Nevertheless, one may still ask: how is it that models that meet the requirements of a symbolic computational theory of mental processes can give rise to fundamental concepts of a theoretical paradigm—such as the connectionist paradigm—which seems to contradict significantly the Fodorian theory? The answer lies in the universal significance of the concept of the network, which lends itself to representing the fundamental structures of different and even conflicting paradigms, which simply adopt different interpretations (Pessa, Penna 1994; Penna, Pessa 1998).

However, this emphasis on the internal state of mental processes (proper to cognitivism) was not without its own inherent problems. Despite its limitations, behaviorism rightly pointed out that internal representations are not easily accessible to objective analysis. Cognitive scientists, in fact, had to come to grips with the harsh reality that internal representations of mental processes corresponded to theoretical constructions, which can hardly be analyzed from an experimental point of view (Squire, Kandel, 2009). The determination of reaction times, for example, allowed scientists to obtain information about the sequence in which these mental operations were being carried out. However, these techniques analyzed the mental representations indirectly and therefore they did not allow researchers to discover how to identify an operation, or to determine to what, exactly, it corresponded. Therefore, in order to make the study of the brain accessible, cognitive psychology had to join forces with biology, which had not been sufficiently taken into consideration by behaviorists. In the second half of the twentieth century, a real revolution occurred in biology as well, which would soon help to arouse keen interest in biologists for the research topics of cognitive psychology. This radical change had two main components that played an important role in the understanding of cognitive processes, especially that of memory: one systemic, the other molecular.

The molecular aspect of the so called biological revolution has its roots, at the turn of the nineteenth and twentieth centuries, on the one hand, in the pioneering works of Mendel, Bateson and Morgan, thanks to whom we know that information that is inherited is passed down from parents to children through genes, that is, discrete biological units located in filamentary structures called chromosomes, contained in the cell nucleus and, on the other hand, in Watson and Crick's discovery in 1953 of the double helix structure of DNA, that double-stranded molecule that constitutes chromosomes and that contains the genetic patrimony in all living beings. This discovery allowed researchers, for the first time in the history of Western philosophical thinking, to offer an adequate, and in a certain sense definitive, answer to the historical diatribe between innatism and empiricism. With the discovery of DNA and of where it resides, innatism won a definitive victory over empiricism, because for the first time the origin of those innate faculties had been identified, which were at the base of any experiential learning and of any form of cognitive process. It was a question, in other words, not of abstract, fixed and unchanging rules, but of rules "incarnated" in a "biochemical language" and able to regulate themselves continually, changing themselves in relation to their environment.

Thus began, in the history of biology, a fascinating adventure connected with the opening of a new frontier regarding the possibility of "dialoguing" with the mystery of human identity and of life in general, through the discovery and decoding of a language that was not of a physical/digital nature (like those of computer theory regarding signals), but of a biochemical nature (natural information): the language of DNA. Thus was born molecular biology, founded on Watson and Crick's discovery, which later gave rise to the "central dogma" of biology: DNA produces RNA which in turn produces the proteins that in turn produce the organism. The DNA of the genes contains a code—the "genetic code"—that is read when the two strands of the DNA double helix separate. Later, one of the two strands is copied, or transcribed, in a complementary RNA copy, called messenger RNA (mRNA). This process is called transcription, since the language of the genes is maintained in the form of a series of adjacent molecules, called nucleotides. Instead, the conversion of mRNA into protein results in the translation from one language, that of nucleotides that correspond to the constituent units of genes and messengers, into another, that of amino acids, which form the constituent units of proteins. Thus, towards the end of the Seventies it became possible to read genetic code sequences and locate the protein encoded by a specific gene. It was thus learned that certain identical DNA fragments encode typically recognizable protein domains or regions. Although those domains are shared by many different proteins, they mediate the same biological function. Knowing the coding sequence of a gene, it became therefore possible to identify certain aspects of the encoded protein's function. A simple comparison of the sequences allowed them to identify the relationship between proteins that carried out their function in different contexts: in different cells of the body of a particular organism or even in very different organisms. As a result, there quickly emerged a general outline of the cell's operation and, in particular, of the way in which cells communicate with each other, which offered a common conceptual framework for understanding many biological processes.

Molecular biology demands our attention even more than quantum mechanics or cosmology—other fields of science affected by a far-reaching revolution in the twentieth century—because it directly affects our daily lives, and is also at the heart of our identity, of who we are. This common structure has already had a major impact on the study of learning in simple invertebrate animals, like the sea slug *Aplysia*, the fruit fly *Drosophila* and the nematode *C. elegans*, which have proved important in the study of behavior. This same pattern is also beginning to allow researchers to study, at the molecular level, the internal representation of cognitive processes in more complex vertebrate animals, including mice (Byrne *et al.*, 1974, 1978; Carew, Pinsker, Kandel 1972). The second aspect of the biological revolution, the systemic one, seeks to associate the elements involved in cognitive function with specific neural dynamics. This task is carried out through the development, as we saw in the previous chapter, of powerful study methods of internal representation of cognitive processes such as Positron Emission Tomography (PET) and Functional Magnetic Resonance Imaging (fMRI).

The systemic neurosciences study neural systems, including those involving vision, memory and language. Neural systems have a certain number of properties in common, including the capacity to process complex information about the environment and about an organism's biological needs. In the human being, this information often reaches consciousness. The systemic neurosciences, therefore, attempt to identify the neural structures and events linked with various steps of the hierarchical process of information processing. The central questions of this field of research regard: thus, how information is encoded (sensory processing); interpreted, thus giving it meaning (perception), stored or modified (learning and memory); used to make predictions about future conditions of one's surroundings and the consequences of one's actions (self-control and emotions); and, used to guide behavior and communicate (language) (Albright *et al.*, 2009).

In this scientific spirit, the fundamental contribution of American psychiatrist Eric Kandel is clearly felt, from the mid-1970s onwards. Kandel is the Nobel Laureate in medicine for 2000 and founder of the Center for Neurobiology and Behavior at Columbia University in New York, where he teaches, and is also chief researcher at the Howard Hughes Medical Institute. His influence is most evident in regard to the study of the molecular basis of synaptic plasticity in the central nervous system in relation to cognitive functions. Studying simple forms of learning in *Aplysia* at the cellular and molecular level, and complementing this approach with molecular genetics and extending it to various forms of learning in mice, the U.S. scientist gave birth to research concerning long-term synaptic plasticity in relation to learning and memory. Kandel especially, by highlighting the close relationship between behaviorist psychology, cognitive psychology, computer science, computability theory and neurophysiology, as well as molecular biology, systemic biology, cognitive neuroscience and the new brain imaging technologies, offers contemporary science of mind the possibility of building a new paradigm and locating a code for it. By placing cognitive psychology and neuroscience in close contact with molecular biology, the great psychiatrist is laying the foundations for the creation of a molecular biology of cognitive activities that in recent years has allowed us to explore on a molecular level mental processes such as the way we think, feel sensations, learn and remember. Kandel's discoveries are manifold. As we shall see in more detail in the next paragraphs, he has provided the first direct evidence that learning changes the effectiveness of specific synapses and that memory depends on the persistence of these modifications. In addition, the fruitful integration promoted by the great scholar between biology and neuro-psychoanalysis, has had a tremendous following in the international scientific community. If, on the one hand, compelling new molecular properties of nerve cells, especially regarding their connections, are continually being discovered thanks to the studies on learning (these results point the way to explaining how nerve connections change during learning and how these changes are maintained over time in the form of memory), on the other hand, the systems of neuroscience and the cognitive sciences are providing information related to how nerve cells collaborate within the neuronal circuits, the organization of learning processes and mnemonic systems and how they work together. In addition, studies of brain and behavioral systems constitute a guide for molecular research, a kind of map that identifies the components of memory and the brain areas in which these components can be studied in greater detail. Many molecular mechanisms, in fact, have come to light since certain nerve cells of specific neuronal circuits could be analyzed while keeping in mind a certain form of memory (Squire, 2004). From a cognitive point of view, on the other hand, cellular and molecular approaches have allowed scientists to glimpse answers to some unresolved questions of the psychology of memory: for example, what changes occur in the brain when we learn and when we remember? Where are memories stored? What is the molecular relationship between the storage of non-declarative memory and that of declarative memory? How are different types of short-term memory related to various forms of long-term memory? In a passage of his speech at the Nobel Foundation in December 2000 Kandel expressed himself thus:

> One of the most remarkable aspects of an animal's behavior is the ability to modify that behavior by learning, an ability that reaches its highest form in human beings. For me, learning and memory have proven to be endlessly fascinating mental processes because they address one of the fundamental features of human activity: our ability to acquire new ideas from experience and to retain these ideas over time in memory. Moreover, unlike other mental processes such as thought, language, and consciousness, learning seemed from the outset to be readily accessible to cellular and molecular analysis. [. . .] My purpose in translating questions about the psychology of learning into the empirical language of biology was not to replace the logic of psychology or psychoanalysis with the logic of cellular molecular biology, but to try to join these two disciplines and to contribute to a new synthesis that would combine the mentalist psychology of memory storage with the biology of neuronal signaling. I hoped further [. . .] that the study of memory storage might reveal new aspects of neuronal signaling. Indeed, this has proven true (Kandel, 2005, pp. 341–342).

In light of all this, therefore, the molecular approaches today are allowing us to place in close relationship the behavior of whole animals with the molecular mechanisms that are carried out in individual cells. Therefore, psychological constructs of the past such as, for example, association, learning, memory storage and remembering can now be addressed in terms of cellular and molecular mechanisms and from a standpoint of brain circuits and systems (Kandel, 2006). In this way we can obtain more accurate information about fundamental processes such as learning and memory.

However, until the mid-twentieth century, many psychologists did not believe that memory could be regarded as a function independent of perception, language or motion. The main reason for this doubt was the fact that the preservation of memory affects many regions of the brain (Kandel *et al.*, 2000). We now know, however, that the hypothesis of widely distributed mnemonic storage need not imply that all brain regions involved in memory functions are equally involved in memory storage. Based on the current vision, memory is widely distributed, with different regions storing different aspects of the whole. Within these areas the redundancy and duplication of functions are scarce. Particular areas possess specific brain functions, and each of these contributes differently to overall memory storage (Squire, Kandel, 2009). Much convincing evidence on the relevance of the temporal lobes for memory were provided in the second half of the twentieth century by the study of patients who had undergone bilateral removal of the hippocampus and surrounding areas of the temporal lobe for the treatment of epilepsy. The first case, and the most renowned one, of the effects on memory caused by the bilateral removal of a part of the temporal lobe was that of the patient H.M. studied by Milner (1966), the Canadian psychologist whose merit it is to have discovered the role of the medial temporal lobe in human memory.[9]

From studies on this patient Milner deduced four fundamental principles:[10] In first place, acquisition of new memories corresponds to a specific brain function, located in the medial portion of the temporal lobes of the brain, and is distinguishable from other perceptual and cognitive capacities. Therefore, the brain's perceptual and intellectual functions are separate from its ability to store data that arise normally from the execution of perceptual and intellectual exercises. Secondly, the medial temporal lobes are not essential to immediate memory. Thirdly, the medial temporal lobe and hippocampus cannot be the ultimate seat of long term memory storage of previously acquired facts.[11] Finally, Milner identified a type of memory that did not depend on the medial temporal lobe (Squire, Kandel, 2009). In the 1962 article titled "Les troubles de la memoire accompagnant des lesions hippocampiques bilaterales," the Canadian psychologist made known the discovery that H.M.'s inability to convert short-term memory into long-term memory was relative. In fact, during an experiment, Milner saw that H.M. was able to learn how to draw the outline of a star by observing the reflection of his hand in a mirror and that his performance improved gradually exactly as in a normal individual. However, each day before starting the experiment, H.M. stated that he had never performed the exercise above. Such studies (Squire, 1987; Squire, Zola-Morgan, 1991; Squire, 2009) marked the beginning of a series of experimental works that would finally permit scholars to identify the biological mechanisms at the base of the two main types of memory. It is not currently known how many different mnemonic systems exist and how these should be named. Nevertheless, there is a widely shared opinion regarding mnemonic systems and the main brain areas most involved in each of these systems (Kandel, 2009; Strata, Thach, Ottersen, 2009). Alternative classification schemes are based simply on different denominations of the same types of memory. The memories for events and motor skills, in fact, are known as registered and unregistered memory, explicit and implicit memory or declarative and non-declarative memory, or procedural, memory (Squire, 1987, 1992).

For simplicity in this paper we will use only one of these terminologies. Damage to the hippocampus and temporal medial lobe, as in the case of H.M., affects declarative memory, while other forms of memory, which have remained intact, will be referred to collectively as non-declarative memory. Declarative memory is the memory for those pieces of information that can be brought to a conscious level in the form of a verbal proposition or as a visual image (for facts, ideas and events). This is the type of memory commonly referred to when using the term "memory": the memory of a person's name, or of the breakfast we had this morning, and so on. Declarative memory can be studied both in humans and animals (Squire, Kandel, 2009). Non-declarative memory also comes from experience, but is expressed in the form of behavioral change and not as mental recall. Unlike declarative memory, non-declarative is unconscious. Non-declarative learning is often accompanied by a certain capacity of recall. We can learn a motor task and then be able to remember a few things about it. We can, for example, imagine ourselves performing the task in question. "Different forms of non-declarative memory are thought to depend on different brain regions, such as the amygdala, the cerebellum, and the striatum, as well as on specific sensory and motor systems recruited for reflexive tasks. Nondeclarative memory may be the only kind of memory available to invertebrate animals because they do not have the brain structures and brain organization that could support declarative memory. They do not, for example, have a hippocampus (Squire, Kandel, 2009, p. 17). Ultimately, according to studies made in the field of biology of cognitive activities, the events that take place in the brain depend on changes in signals between individual neurons, and these, in turn, depend on the activity of particular molecules present in nerve cells. Following the line of research established by Kandel and Squire, therefore, we may ask whether these two distinct forms of memory use different molecular events to deposit the memory, or whether it involves fundamentally similar mechanisms. How does short-term storage differ from long-term? Perhaps the two types of storage take place in different locations, or perhaps a single neuron can store information pertaining to both the short-term and long-term memory?

2.2 Synaptic plasticity and non-declarative memory

The thought of studying the molecular mechanisms of memory storage at first sight seems amazing, almost utopian. It is estimated that the brain of a mammal is composed of about a hundred billion nerve cells and connections between these cells are many times more numerous (Kandel *et al.*, 2000). How, then, in this extraordinarily large population of cells, could we ever locate those involved in memory storage?

Fortunately, the task of identifying the molecular mechanisms that take place inside the cells can be simplified through experiments. Today, in fact, scientists are able to study forms of memory storage that involve only a few restricted portions of the entire nervous system of vertebrates, such as the spinal cord, the cerebellum, the amygdala and the hippocampus. Even more radically, it is possible to analyze the much simpler nervous system of invertebrate animals. As regards the study of the latter, it is sometimes possible to identify individual nerve cells directly involved in a particular type of learning. In this way it is possible to identify the molecular changes that take place inside the neurons responsible for learning and memory storage.

This experimental approach began between 1957 and 1960, with studies by Kandel on hippocampal cell properties conducted at the National Institutes of Health in Bethesda during his post-doctoral fellowship (Kandel, Spencer, 1961). In those years the young Viennese scholar began to abandon the psychological approach to the study of memory in favor of the biological approach, in order to understand how learning changes the neural networks of the brain. But while Kandel attempted to translate the topics of the psychology of learning into the empirical language of biology, he did not do so to replace the psychological or psychoanalysis theories with molecular and cellular explanations, but to try to bring these two disciplines into dialogue, while contributing in an equally decisive way to the creation of a new theoretical synthesis capable of keeping together the mentalist psychology of memory and the biology of neural signals. He moreover rightly believed that the study of the biological bases of memory would help illumine other matters pertaining to the signaling properties of neurons (Kandel, 1998, 1999).

Kandel started out wondering, somewhat naively, whether the electrophysiological properties of hippocampal pyramidal cells, considered essential for memory, were fundamentally different from other neurons of the brain. During his research, it became apparent that all nerve cells, including pyramidal ones, have similar signaling properties (Kandel, Spencer, 1968). Thus, the unique functions of the hippocampus had to derive not so much from the inherent properties of the pyramidal cells, but rather from the network of functional interconnections between the latter and the various forms of learning. However, it remained to be discovered how the sensory information regarding the task of learning reached the hippocampus, thus prompting the behavioral response. The undertaking was not a simple one, since the hippocampus has many neurons and countless interconnections. To exploit the potential of the tools of biology in the study of learning, Kandel adopted "a radical reductionist approach": "We needed to study not the most complex but the simplest instances of memory storage, and to study them in animals that were most tractable experimentally. Such a reductionist approach was hardly new in twentieth-century biology." (Kandel, 2005, p. 343). In the middle of the twentieth century, when it came to studying behavior, many biologists were reluctant to adopt this reductionist strategy. The same thing was true for psychologists, who rejected the idea that learning could be reduced to an area of biology in which the use of simple animal models, especially those of invertebrates, could have a good chance of success. On the contrary, they believed that only higher animals showed interesting forms of learning and that these required an organization and a qualitatively different neural apparatus than those observed in simpler organisms. Instead, Kandel believed their concerns about the use of a simple experimental apparatus to study learning were unfounded: "If elementary forms of learning are common to all animals with an evolved nervous system, the mechanisms of learning at the cell and molecular level must retain features that can be studied effectively even in simple invertebrate animals" (p. 343). In Kandel's opinion, the suitable animal for this kind of experimental study was the giant sea snail *Aplysia* for some fundamental reasons. First, its nervous system is composed of a limited number of cells; many of these are huge and many have unique characteristics that make them easily recognizable to a naked eye (Frazier *et al.*, 1967; Kandel, 1976). Second, *Aplysia*'s neurons can be easily dissected in biochemical studies, so it is possible to collect enough mRNA from a single cell to construct a whole library of cDNA (Kandel, 2007). Third, it is possible to inject markers, genetic constructs or antibodies smoothly into these cells; these procedures have allowed the molecular study of signal transduction in isolated neurons (Kandel, 2001). By virtue of these elements, the great psychiatrist was able to describe a very simple defensive reflex: gill retraction in response to stimulation of the siphon, a response similar to that of a hand retracting quickly from the hot water. If one applies a light tactile stimulus to the siphon, both it and the gill retract into the cavity of the mantle, seeking protection under its fold (Pinsker *et al.*, 1970).

In studies by Pinsker and Kupfermann and later by Kandel, Hawkins and Carew, it was shown that this simple reflex can be changed using three different forms of learning, i.e. sensitization, habituation and classical conditioning (Carew, Pinsker, Kandel, 1972; Pinsker *et al.*, 1973). Sensitization and habituation are examples of non-associative learning, where a subject learns the properties of a single stimulus when repeatedly exposed to it. In contrast, classical and operative conditioning are examples of associative learning: in this case the subject learns the relationship between two stimuli (classical conditioning) or between a stimulus and a behavioral response (instrumental conditioning and operative conditioning). In the 1950s, behaviorist psychologists had focused their efforts on these forms of learning, but focusing solely on the acquisition of knowledge, rather than on its storage, they failed to recognize (and in fact they were not very interested in recognizing) that the memory of non-declarative knowledge was an unconscious process. In addition, by treating non-declarative cognition as a model for the acquisition of any kind of knowledge, the behaviorists basically ignored what today we call declarative memory (Squire, Kandel, 2009).

With the experimental studies inspired by the new methodological reductionism proposed by Kandel and other scholars, it has been possible to highlight some deep cerebral processes which are at the basis of transmission mechanisms and information storage. In fact, one of the discoveries of the modern molecular biology of cognitive activity is that a single connection between two neurons constitutes a basic unit of memory storage. The 10^{14} connections in the human encephalon provide therefore a rough indication of our maximum storage capacity of information (Squire, Kandel, 2009). The nervous signaling process often begins with physical events in the surrounding environment that affect our body. "The surprising fact about neuronal signals is that they are remarkably stereotypical. Nerve signals that convey visual information are identical to those that carry information about sounds or odors. In turn, the incoming signals that carry sensory information into the nervous system are similar to the outgoing signals that convey the commands for movement" (Squire, Kandel, 2009, p. 31). The fact that the nature of the information conveyed by nervous input is not determined by the nature of this signal, but the particular path followed by the same signal within the encephalon, is one of the milestone of brain functions.[12] The brain receives codes and interprets patterns of electrical signals that reach it through specific pathways and in this way processes visual information in a particular group of nerve circuits and auditory information in another set of circuits.[13] The first studies on the relationships between single nervous cells and the encephalon as a whole began thanks to the brilliant insights of Ramon y Cayal (1894, 1911), who was the first to understand the signaling mechanisms of the encephalon and the hypothesis on the synaptic changing. Such studies awarded the great Spanish scientist, in 1937, the Nobel Prize for Physiology.

Unlike his contemporaries, he was able to go beyond a simple anatomical description of the neurons. In fact, the Spanish scholar had the amazing ability to observe a static structure and to deduce information from that observation, related to the structure's function. He intuited, for instance, that the four anatomical portions of the neuron had different roles in the transmission of signals. Based on this fact, Ramon y Cayal (1894, 1911) formulated the idea that neurons were "dynamically polarized," i.e., that within each nerve cell the information flowed in a predetermined and constant direction (Kandel, 2006). The nerve cell receives signals at the dendrites and cell body and from these reception areas the information is conveyed to the axon and presynaptic terminals. Later experimental studies have confirmed this hypothesis. In the first half of the twentieth Century, researchers managed to demonstrate that neurons used two signals: a) stereotyped "action potentials," based on the principle of all-or-nothing, to transfer information from one compartment to another of the neuron and b) different levels of "synaptic potentials" to transmit the information from one nerve cell to another by means of a process known as synaptic transmission (Squire, Kandel, 2009).

The action potential is an electric signal to depolarize, transmitted from dendrites to the cell body and all along the axon to the presynaptic terminals, where the neuron is in contact with other nerve cells (Squire, Kandel, 2009; Tempia, Bravin, Strata, 1996). Ramón y Cajal understood that neurons communicate with each other at the synapses level. While the axon signal, the action potential, is a constant signal of considerable size, based on the principle of all-or-nothing, the synapse signal, the so-called synaptic potential, comes in various strengths and can be modified.[14] The current produced by the action potential in the presynaptic cell can't just jump through the synaptic gap to activate the postsynaptic target cell. At the level of the synapse, rather, the signal undergoes a transformation. When the action potential reaches the presynaptic terminal, the electric signal causes the release of a chemical (neurotransmitter) which is poured into the synaptic cleft, where it acts as a signal for the target cell.[15] However, chemical input is not only related to chemical neurotransmitters or nerve cells of the encephalon, but constitutes a "universal communication mechanism," used by all cells of living systems.[16]

Today we know that the formation of nerve networks relies on a complex framework of distributed interconnected programs able to regulate gene expression over the entire course of a human being's development (Fox, Keller, 2010). The presence of such precise nerve circuits presents us with a fundamental question: when we learn or remember, the nerve cells presumably undergo some kind of change, but if the connections between neurons are arranged so rigorously, in what, then, does this modification consist? Thanks to a remarkable intuition, Ramón y Cajal proposed an answer to this dilemma. In a famous 1894 article entitled: "*The croonian lecture: la fine structure des centers nerveux,*" formulated the hypothesis, now known as "synaptic plasticity hypothesis," according to which the "strength of synaptic connections," is not a fixed property, but is "modifiable," "plastic," namely synaptic strength could be modified by neuronal activity. Arguing that the process of learning that could constitute brain activity, Ramon and Cajal saw that, thanks to this altered activity, the changed neurons would be able to modulate their own communication skills. Thus, it was established that the basic mechanism of memory storage is founded in that functional property (synaptic plasticity) that is the expression of the persistence of those alterations in synaptic communication (Ramon y Cajal 1894; Kandel, Squire, 2009).

Similarly to what happened with the first suggestions for mnemonic systems, these brilliant insights were ignored for about half a century by the scientific community—which meanwhile debated alternative theories—as they were deemed unsatisfactory because of their lack of experimental evidence. It was therefore necessary, over the course of the ensuing decades, to study simple nervous systems of organisms in order to examine the connections directly, during learning. Only in this way would it be possible to find out whether memory storage was actually based on changes in the strength of the connections between nerve cells (Squire, 2004, 2007).[17]

Kandel, Kupfermann, Castellucci, Carew and Hawkins subjected many theories to direct verification, trying to understand how there could be learning in a neural circuit characterized by pre-fixed elements. To address the issue Kandel and his colleagues examined the neural circuit of the retraction reflex of *Aplysia*'s gill in a condition of sensitization, classical conditioning or habituation (Kandel 1976, 1978; Castellucci, Kandel, 1974). In the course of their studies, these scientists identified many cells of the gill's retraction network.[18] Once researchers had identified the individual cells of the neural circuit, they were able to confront the problem concerning the way in which learning and memory storage carried out in a nerve network. Noting the pattern of connections of the gill-withdrawal reflex is set once and for all early in development, while the precise strength of the connections is not. Thus, Castellucci, Kandel and colleagues studied the synaptic depression at the junction between a sensory neuron and a motor neuron (Castellucci *et al.*, 1970; Kupfermann, 1970; Castellucci *et al.*, 1978, 1980; Pinskey et al. 1970, 1973). They observed that depending on the number of training sessions, where 10 stimuli were applied to the sensory neuron, the synaptic depression can persist for a period of time ranging from several minutes to several hours (and, as we shall see shortly, even longer), but still persists for exactly the same time period of the behavioral habituation. As soon as the synapses return to their original strength, the animal starts to respond to stimulation of the siphon with a rapid retraction of the gill and siphon. Ramón y Cayal's hypotheses thus found their experimental corroboration. It was evident that learning depends on changes in the efficacy of synaptic connections between precisely interconnected cells.

Therefore, such studies have highlighted numerous general principles of memory storage. Firstly, they have provided the first direct evidence that the synaptic connections between neurons are not stable, but can be modified as a result of learning and these changes in synaptic strength persist and are a basic component of memory storage. Secondly, we know today what causes changes in the strength of the connections between two crucial groups of neurons involved in retraction of the gill reflex (motor neurons and sensory neurons) and that these changes are based on alteration in presynaptic terminals and in particular on modifications in the number of synaptic vesicles released. Even though it was later shown that numerous other plastic mechanisms contribute to memory storage, changing the amount of neurotransmitter released has proven to be a very common mechanism in the generation of memory in many systems like this. Thirdly, in the gill's retraction reflex, a reduction in synaptic strength does not involve only the synapses between the sensory neurons and their target cells, but also occurs in the synapses of interneurons and target cells. Even the storage of a simple non-declarative memory is distributed over multiple locations. "Finally, the findings illustrate that non-declarative memory storage does not depend on specialized 'memory' neurons, whose only function is to store information. Rather, the capability for simple nondeclarative memory storage is built directly into the synapses connecting the neurons that make up the neural circuit of the behavior being modified. Memory storage results from changes in neurons that are themselves components of the reflex pathway. Thus, the remembrance of the habituation is embedded in the same neuronal circuit that produces the behavior" (Squire, Kandel, 2009, p. 46). In this sense, as we will see later taking into consideration the reflections of Kandel, Squire and Damasio, non-declarative memory differs from declarative memory, in which a whole neuronal system, located in the medial temporal lobe, is designated to help impress the memories of past events. So far we have focused more on short-term memory, memory that lasts for a few minutes. We will now look in more detail at long-term memory, which may persist throughout life, deepening the molecular aspects of learning and cognition.

2.3 The molecular biology of short-term and long-term memory

In this paragraph we will focus on the molecular mechanisms that govern the consolidation of short-term memory and in which way the transition to long-term memory occurs. Kandel, in collaboration with Schwartz, to address the issue, started from short-term sensitization and discovered that changes at the synaptic level, as well as their short-term response, appeared even when protein synthesis was inhibited, suggesting that short-term synaptic plasticity could be mediated by a second messenger system cyclic AMP (cAMP) (Schwartz *et al.*, 1971). Kandel, Schwartz and Cedar, continuing their experiments on *Aplysia* discovered that electrical stimulation of the modulatory pathways involved in facilitating heterosynaptic modulators induces an increase in cAMP in the abdominal ganglion and that the likely neurotransmitters at play here (serotonin and dopamine) could simulate the effects of electrical stimulation and increase cAMP levels. Kandel, Hawkins and other scholars described the modulatory system, activated by a stimulus-sensitizer on the tail (Hawkins *et al.*, 1981), confirming that it contains serotonergic interneurons. Kandel and colleagues subsequently found that serotonin "acts on specific receptors in the presynaptic terminals of the sensory neuron" (Kandel, 2005), which causes the enhancement of neurotransmitter release. The scientists observed, also, a presynaptic facilitation when they injected CAMP directly into presynaptic cells (Kandel *et al.*, 1976). This offered one of the first experimental evidence regarding the involvement of cAMP in the control of synaptic efficacy, which gave them the first data on one of the molecular mechanisms of short-term memory: the regulation of neurotransmitter release.

Having reached this point in their research, Kandel and his colleagues directed their studies towards an attempt to understand how cAMP increased the quantity of neurotransmitter released, and they realized that serotonin, or the administering of cAMP, increases the excitability and extends the action potential by reducing the K^+ currents, thus allowing a greater flow of Ca^{2+} in the presynaptic terminal at every action potential (Klein, Kandel, 1980). Taking up one of Greengard's ideas, who had advanced the hypothesis that cAMP acts in the brain via the PKA (cAMP-dependent protein-kinase A), Kandel and Klein argued that cAMP could cause the phosphorylation of this K^+ channel precisely by activating PKA. In the same year, in a series of experiments it was discovered that the active catalytic sub-unit of PKA alone produces an extension of the action potential, and an increase of glutamate released by the terminal (Castellucci *et al.*, 1980) and that, vice versa, the specific peptide that inhibits PKA (PKI) blocks the action of serotonin. These results have provided direct evidence of the role of PKA in short-term presynaptic facilitation. Finally, Kandel and, independently, Byrne and his collaborators have shown that serotonin increases the amount of neurotransmitter released that not only increases the action potential, but even acts on the release mechanisms, in ways that are not yet known. In other words, "serotonin leads to increase in presynaptic cAMP, which activates PKA" and strengthens the synapses through an increase in neurotransmitter, favored by a combination of processes (Kandel, 2001).

By administering serotonin (a neurotransmitter released by *Aplysia* when it receives a shock to its tail) instead of the shock itself, Montarolo, Kandel and other scholars studied the sensitization in a prepared culture made up of a single sensory cell that formed synaptic connections with a single motor neuron (Montarolo *et al.*, 1986). The scholars were thus able to induce facilitation, in both the short- and long-term, noting that, as also occurs in healthy animals, the long-term process differs from the short-term in that it requires the synthesis of new proteins.[19] Starting from this cell culture, the scientists wondered: which genes regulate the transition from the short-term to the long-term process, and which ones are essential for the consolidation of the latter? Kandel and colleagues observed that five applications of serotonin, at intervals (instead of five shocks to the tail) will activate PKA, which in turn activates a mitogen-activated protein kinase (MAPK). Both translocate into the nucleus, where they trigger a transcriptional cascade process from the transcription factor CREB-1 (cAMP response element-binding protein-1), so called because it binds the cAMP responsive elements (CRE) in the promoters of target genes (Kandel, 2001)[20]. As shown by Bailey and Chen (1988, 1989), long-term memory depends on the development of new synaptic connections, a structural change that occurs parallel to the continuation of the response. With the fading of memory, the connections unbind. Moreover, as Bartsch discovered in 1995, positive regulators represent only one side of the coin, as the memory is also subject to inhibitory controls. Synaptic facilitation in the long term demands, in fact, not only the activation of genes that promote memory, but also the non-activation of suppressor genes. One of these, the ApCREB-2 transcription factor, can repress the transcription mediated by ApCREB-1a; the removal of this inhibition lowers the threshold of the long term memorization process (Kandel, 2001).

In the light of all this, therefore, long-term memory depends on the initiation of a rigidly controlled, domino-like process of genic activation, in which the suppressor genes of the memory establish a threshold or a point of verification with regard to the process of consolidating the memory, probably in order to ensure that only the salient aspects are learned (Kandel, 2005). Memory suppressants can allow emotionally-charged stimuli to drive the memorization process, as occurs in the so-called "photographic memories"—memories of events with a strong emotional charge that are relived in the minutest detail, as if the full scene were instantly imprinted in the brain.

The discovery of a transcriptional cascade process explains why the long-term memory requires the synthesis of new proteins immediately after training, but poses a new problem of a biological-cellular nature. A single neuron forms hundreds of connections on many different target cells. We know that the synaptic transformations in the short-term regard only specific synapses. But then, considering that the long-term synaptic changes require a transcription process and thus, the intervention of the nucleus, we can ask whether the long-term memory is a process that affects the cell in its entirety, or if rather cellular-biological mechanisms are at work, maintaining the principle of synaptic specificity even in long-term facilitation. In order to deepen the issue, Martin studied in a culture one sensory cell of the *Aplysia* with a branched axon and two motor neurons, joined by two clearly separated synapses (Martin *et al.*, 1998). In this culture, a single application of serotonin to one of the two synapses produced a transient facilitation only in that synapse, as expected. Five applications of serotonin to a branch induce long-term facilitation, which in this case too is limited to the stimulated synapse. This long-term synapse-specific facilitation requires CREB and, moreover, induces structural changes. Despite the nucleus' intervention, therefore, long-term changes in synaptic structure and functioning are confined to the synapses stimulated by serotonin. In an attempt to find an explanation for this, Martin and Kandel noted that five applications of serotonin sends a signal to the nucleus, by activating CREB-1, which in turn sends proteins to all the terminals. However, only the terminals marked by serotonin endings can employ these proteins productively for synaptic growth. In fact, one application of serotonin is sufficient to mark the synapse, causing it to intercept, albeit in reduced form, the long-term facilitation induced in the other site by five applications of serotonin (Kandel, 2001).

Given this situation, Kandel writes:

> These results gave us a new and surprising insight into short-term facilitation. The stimulus that produces the short-term process has two functions [...]. When acting alone, it provides a selective, synapse-specific enhancement of synaptic strength, which contributes to short-term memory, lasting minutes. When acting in conjunction with the activation of CREB initiated by a long-term process in either that synapse or in any other synapse on the same neuron, the stimulus locally marks those synapses at which it occurs. The marked synapse can then utilize the proteins activated by CREB for synaptic growth to produce a persistent change in synaptic strength. Thus, the logic for the long-term process involves a long-range integration that is different from the short-term process. In the long-term, a synapse's function is determined not only by the history of usage of that synapse, it is also determined by the state of the transcriptional machinery in the nucleus" (Kandel, 2001, pp. 134–135).

Thus, for the structural changes to last, the synthesis of proteins is required *in situ*. Steward's decisive contribution showed that dendrites contain ribosomes, after, and that particular mRNA are transported to the dendrites and translated there (Steward, 1997). Further, Kandel's experiments showed that one function of these mRNA translated *in situ* is to stabilize the functional and structural changes in the short term relating to specific synapses. Such research has thus revealed a fourth type of synaptic action (mediated by the signals of the neurotransmitters) constituted by the marking of the synapse and the adjustment of the localized synthesis of proteins, which contributes to the consolidation of long-term synapse-specific facilitation.[21] Overall, these studies have made it possible to understand the reasons why the synapses are so versatile and effective for the purposes of memory storage. They have a variety of molecular mechanisms able to persist in their activities for shorter or longer periods and can increase or decrease the amount of transmitter released after the arrival of an action potential. A single type of synapse can store many different types of memory. These results have an important philosophical implication at the level of philosophy of biology. "The cAMP pathway is not unique to memory storage. It is not even unique to neurons, as it is used in many other cells of the body [. . .] in order to produce persistent action. In fact, of all known second-messenger systems, the cAMP system is probably the most primitive and is conserved through the course of evolutionary history. It is the only major second messenger system found in primitive single-celled organisms like bacteria, where it serves as a system to signal hunger. Thus, memory storage mechanisms in the brain did not evolve through the creation of a specialized set of molecules. Memory does not use a special, memory related second-messenger system. Rather, memory has co-opted an efficient signaling system that is used for *other* purposes in *other* cells" (Squire, Kandel, 2009, pp. 58–59). The biochemical language of memory shows, in fact, that general biological principle. Evolution does not create new and specific molecules whenever a new and specialized function evolves, but, as pointed out by the French biologist Jacob, evolution works rather like "a tinkerer who uses everything at his disposal to produce some kind of workable object" (Jacob, 1977, p. 1163). Evolution always uses the same set of slightly modified genes. It creates variations (new functions) thanks to the generation of random changes (mutations) in the genetic structure, which give rise to slightly different variants of a protein (Jacob, 1982, 1983). According to Darwin most mutations are neutral or even harmful and they are not maintained. Only in rare cases they increase an individual's ability to survive and to reproduce. These latter are those that have the most chance of being maintained over time. Therefore, a new function is carried out by existing and slightly modified molecules or new combinations of existing proteins. In his 1977 article entitled: "Evolution and Tinkering," Jacob describes this feature of evolution as follows: "What distinguishes a butterfly from a lion, a hen from a fly, or a worm from a whale is much less a difference in chemical constituents than in the organization and the distribution of these constituents. The few big steps of evolution required acquisition of new information. But specialization and diversification occurred by using differently the same structural information. Among neighboring groups, vertebrates for instance, chemistry is the same. What makes one vertebrate different from another is a change in the time of expression and in the relative amounts of gene products rather than the small differences observed in the structure of these products. It is a matter of regulation rather than of structure. [. . .] Small changes modifying the distribution in time and space of the same structures are sufficient to affect deeply the form, the functioning and the behavior of the final product—the adult animal. It is always a matter of using the same elements, of adjusting them, of altering here or there, of arranging various combinations to produce new objects of increasing complexity. It is always a matter of tinkering" (Jacob, 1977, p. 1165).

Now, seen from the perspective of the various forms of learning, synaptic plasticity emerges, then, as a complex dialectic process of generation, transmission and assimilation of information within the nervous system and between the latter and the external environment, meaning a "tinkering" process, namely, that has its roots in the very molecular structure of chemical synapses, and, more generally, in the teleonomic performance of their proteins. In this respect, let us close this section with a reference to the brilliant insights of Monod, one of the fathers of molecular biology and of the genetic code, who by placing cybernetics, developmental biology and biochemistry in close conjunction, starting from the 1960s, highlighted the similarities between automata and self-controlled natural systems, also developing a mechanistic model of the molecular and cognitive processes of living organisms. Contemporary experimental research on the biochemical mechanisms of the transmission of information, as we have seen, only confirms the Monodian doctrine of the gratuity of the cellular processes that, in 1970, in one of the most important pages of *Chance and Necessity* he summarizes thus: "The organism is a self-constructing machine. Its macroscopic structure is not imposed upon it by outside forces. It shapes itself autonomously by dint of constructive internal interactions. Although our understanding of the mechanisms of development is still very imperfect, we can from now on state that the constructive interactions are microscopic and molecular, and that the molecules involved are essentially if not uniquely proteins. Hence they are proteins that channel the activity of the chemical machine, ensure its coherent functioning, and put it together. All these teleonomic performances rest, in the final analysis, upon the proteins' so-called 'stereospecific' properties, that is to say upon their ability to 'recognize' other molecules (including other proteins) by their *shape,* this shape being determined by their molecular structure. There is here, quite literally, a microscopic discriminative (if not 'cognitive') faculty. We may say that any teleonomic performance or structure in a living being—whatever it may be—can, in principle at least, be analyzed in terms of stereospecific interactions involving one, several, or a very large number of proteins" (Monod, 1974, p. 52). It follows then—and this is the key point—that in terms of regulation by the mediation of a protein, anything is possible. "And it is in the structure of these molecules that one must see the ultimate source of the autonomy, or more precisely, the self-determination that characterizes living beings in their behavior" (p. 79). It is, therefore, especially the identification of the notion of gratuity (understood as the arbitrariness of cellular processes) that characterizes the conceptual approach of Monodian research; biological instructions, in fact, essentially constitute a message, that is, they are not bound to a kind of necessary chemical relationship with the molecules that "interpret" them. With the same DNA bases, it is possible to compose different messages and similar proteins can perform many different actions, given the appropriate context. Regulatory systems direct cell activity, thus making them a functional unit. The analysis of synaptic interactions demonstrates how a single protein molecule is already capable of regulating its activity on the basis of a multiplicity of chemical information. It is clear, then, that the teleonomic activities, both for Monod and for Kandel, are not the exclusive property of complex systems whose order finds its ultimate foundation in the amazing harmony of free chemical interactions. In light of all this, therefore, the activities of neurons without exception are subordinate to each other either directly or indirectly[22]: "On such a basis, but not that of a vague 'general theory of systems,' it becomes possible for us to grasp how in a very real sense the organism effectively transcends physical laws—even while obeying them—thus achieving at once the pursuit and fulfillment of its own purpose" (p. 81).

2.4 Declarative memory and brain systems

Declarative memory consists in calling to mind an event of the past, it is namely the conscious evocation of data. At the beginning of this chapter, we introduced the distinction between two main types of memory, namely, declarative (or explicit) and non-declarative (or implicit) and we underlined how they are dependent upon separate cerebral systems. In this section, we will concentrate our attention on the many, distinct operations of declarative memory such as coding, storage and retrieval and the different brain systems that support its operations. Declarative memory is memory for knowledge that can potentially be declared, i.e., called to mind verbally or in the form of mental images. The fact that something perceived will be remembered later is determined by a number of factors, the most important of which operate around the time of learning: influencing the nature and the extent of the *encoding* of the information, namely on the effectiveness that occurs at the moment in which a new event or a new fact generates neural changes in the brain.

To encode literally means "to convert the information into a code" (Squire, Kandel, 2009, p. 74). Within psychology, the term "encode" is used in this same way to refer to the way the material we come into contact with is handled, processed and prepared to be deposited in the memory. When learning is intentional rather than accidental, this increases the likelihood of having a strong and lasting memory, combining processes of codification with meticulous learning (McDaniel, Thomas, 2007). A role of fundamental importance, at the level of the codification of information under the form of memory, is played therefore, by the biological meaning, that is the capability of the human being to give sense to things through perception. Meaning plays a role of information selector giving to long term memory a capability apparently unlimited. It can hold several thousand facts, concepts and schemas, sometimes for life. In what way, though, does the codified information persist in the form of memory?

To address this issue, according to Squire and Kandel (1996, 2000, 2009), what proved particularly important were studies carried out with functional techniques of image processing on healthy individuals during brain activity. The regions of the cerebral cortex involved in the perception and in the elaboration of colors, sizes, shapes and other objects aspects coincide with the regions involved in memory evocation of these same objects. Although there is no single repository for memory, the latter is, however, not evenly distributed throughout the nervous system. Each region involved in representing a single event contributes differently to the whole representation" (Squire, Kandel, 2009). Squire and Kandel (2009) have defined as an "engram" the total amount of brain changes that initially encoded an experience and that, subsequently, constitute the memory of the same. In principle, the "engram" of a declarative memory is distributed on several brain regions, specialized for particular kinds of assimilation-perception and informational accommodation processing. This principle makes it possible to understand the extraordinary achievements made by individuals who are special experts in a particular field. Such knowledge, however, does not depend on being gifted with exceptional mnemonic skill, but rather on an extremely specialized ability, gained through experience, to encode and organize specific types of information (Squire, 1987).

Let us now examine the workings of recall. Calling to mind an object means collecting diverse information distributed over different areas of the cerebral cortex and reassembling it in such a way as to achieve a coherent whole. The remembering performed here, however, is not a simple reactivation of those multiple fragments variously distributed that constitute the engram. According to the additional stimulus or suggestion available, in many cases only certain parts of the system are activated. If the additional stimulus (the recall signal) is weak or ambiguous, the reactivated memory might even differ from the information stored (Squire, Kandel, 2009). Therefore, a person who remembers is engaged in a complex process of reconstructing past events, and is not performing a simple mental rewind. Finally, a mnemonic experience can be considered accurate and subjectively adequate when in reality it is only an approximation and not an exact reproduction (Kandel *et al.*, 2000). In this sense, Schacter (2001a) stressed the importance of the recall stimuli and the context. Having a good storage memory does not guarantee the certainty of being able to recall these same events properly long after. The mood and the mental state of mind can affect what and how we remember. Retrieval, in fact, is more successful when the context and recall stimuli present when learning correspond to those present when we try to remember what we have learned.[23]

So far we have considered the nature of declarative memory during encoding, storage and recall. Now we'll start to explore, again using the main works of Kandel and Squire, how the brain accomplishes these tasks. At this level of analysis, the interaction between cognitive psychology and systems biology becomes especially evident. "Unlike non-declarative memory, the transformation of a short-term declarative memory into a long-term declarative memory is not only a question of synaptic connections growing stronger in these brain areas. An entirely new brain system comes into play, the medial temporal lobe system. This system is essential for the long-term storage of declarative memory." (Squire, Kandel, 2009, p. 91).

The expression "short-term memory," in its general meaning, refers to those mnemonic processes that hold the information only temporarily, until the memory is forgotten or incorporated into a more stable, long-term and potentially permanent depository. The information, therefore, is what constitutes the center of attention and occupies the current flow of thoughts. Immediate memory capacity (the ability to keep in mind something in an active way from the moment that the information is received) is quite limited and, when the content is not being recalled, its duration is usually less than 30 seconds (Squire, 1992). When, instead, the concepts are being actively recalled, it can be prolonged over time and its contents can persist for several minutes. This temporal extension of immediate memory is known as working memory (Baddeley, Hitch 1974). An object or event is initially represented in immediate memory, but their representation can be supported by working memory and the memory can persist in the form of long-term memory. "Short-term memory," therefore, refers not only to the immediate memory, limited in its capacity, and the recall systems of the working memory, but also to memory components that occur later in reference to the cellular and molecular events that lead to synaptic changes (Kandel, Pittenger, 2003; Kandel, 1989, 1997).

The immediate memory and working memory, therefore, can be imagined as a kind of collection of temporary memory capabilities that operate parallel to each other (Baddeley, 2000, 2004).

No specific test is able to determine the duration of the awareness and ability of a hypothetical repository for all types of working memory. Nevertheless, biologists have begun to understand how temporary memory functions are arranged in the encephalon thanks to neurophysiological studies conducted on monkeys[24]. Experiments conducted on monkeys have shown that during the performance of delayed matching between two objects, are characterized by neuronal activity in the TE area, during the delay the neurons in an area of the frontal cortex were continually active. Buffalo, Zhang, Desimone and colleagues, moreover, pointed out an important difference between the activity in the frontal cortex and that of the temporal lobe during this time frame. These scholars intuited that it was possible to interrupt the activity of the temporal lobe during the delay simply by presenting the animals with additional visual stimuli. In the meantime the neuronal activity in the frontal cortex continued uninterruptedly (Buffalo *et al,* 2010; Zhang *et al.*, 2011).

In such circumstances, according to Squire and Kandel, the delayed activity in the frontal cortex could be particularly important for maintaining information in the working memory, despite the distraction. In fact, injury to the frontal cortex reduces the monkeys' performance in tests on their working memory. It is believed, therefore, that neuronal activity in the TE area signals the impending arrival of sensory information. It is thought that a subsequent feedback "from top to bottom" in the frontal cortex sustains the neuronal activity in sensory areas through a delay, additionally predisposing those areas to important stimuli for the behavior currently underway, which stimuli need to be retained in the working memory (Kandel, 2009; Squire, 2007). "This cognitive control permits memory to be accessed strategically, and orchestrates the use of behavior-guiding rules that allow knowledge relevant to current goals to be brought to mind and put to flexible use. In the absence of these prefrontal regions, individuals are stimulus-bound and able to react only to the immediate sensory environment" (Squire, Kandel, 2009, p. 95).

The process that stores information in long-term memory and, as we shall see, this process depends on particular structures of the medial portion of the temporal lobe. The medial temporal lobe is not however the ultimate depository of long-term memory (Kandel,

Squire, 2000; Kandel, 2009, 2012). One would expect, therefore, that memory could be distributed among area TE in the temporal lobe, area PG in the parietal lobe, and other areas, but in reality are aggregate that happens in these areas changes in the collection of the altered neurons comprise the long-term memory of what was perceived (Squire, Kandel, 2009, p. 96). Further, studies on patients with brain injuries have made it possible to locate the storage of long-term memories. These studies have revealed a surprising degree of specialization within the cerebral cortex and confirm the idea that the storage of different memory types relies on different brain regions in a category-specific manner (Warrington, McCarthy, 1983). Hall, Liu, Martin and colleagues located the brain regions responsible for the storage of category-specific knowledge by using functional magnetic resonance imaging (fRMI) (Hall *et al.*, 2001). In this way it was possible to identify specific cortical areas that undergo increased activity when an individual pronounces the name of an animal compared to when they pronounce the name of a tool, while in other areas the cortical activity increases when the name of a tool is pronounced, rather than the name of an animal. The areas that respond better when you say the name of an animal can be found in the temporal lobe, particularly in the right hemisphere, "In the case of tools, regions are more active in the left hemisphere, specifically in the temporal lobe, parietal cortex and ventral premotor cortex." (Squire, Kandel, 2009, p. 98). Moreover, these results, consonant with those obtained from Warrington and McCarthy on patients with brain lesions, show that the properties of objects, together with their perception and their use, affect the brain area where long-term representations about the identity of these objects come to be stored. Polyn and Norman (2009) have shown that these specialized cortical regions are active not only in perception (when the individual learns concepts relating to a particular category), but also, when the individual recalls these notions at a later time. Therefore, when individuals try to remember the basics of a particular category learned recently, their brain activity progressively resembles that present at the time of learning (Squire, Kandel, 2009).

When any of the areas involved in visual processing is damaged, what follows is specific damage at the level of perception (Kandel, 2001). An important lesson on the neuronal organization of mnemonic functions derives from the observation that, unlike the effects caused by a lesion in the area of visual processing (for example in the lateral temporal lobe), damage to the medial temporal lobe level does not affect perceptual capabilities in any way. However, an injury to this structure results in a much more general defect: all declarative memory is compromised (Kandel et *al.*, 2000; Kandel, 2001). As we saw previously, "memory is a normal consequence of perception. The medial temporal lobe allows for the lasting effects of perceptual experience that we call memory. To transform a visual perception and the immediate memory into a persistent, long-term declarative memory, the medial temporal lobes of the brain must first store aspects of the developing memory. It must then interact with the cortical areas that support perception and immediate memory" (Squire, Kandel, 2009, p. 99).

One of the important characteristics of declarative memory is that an injury to the hippocampal system does not harm learning only, from that moment onwards, but can also affect the memories acquired before the injury. This phenomenon, known as retrograde amnesia, was carefully studied for the first time in the nineteenth century by Ribot. The scholar had noticed that a brain injury or illness at the base of a mnemonic deficit, influenced primarily recent memory, while remote memory tended to be less affected (Ribot, 1887). These observations are today known as Ribot's law according to which the memory loss is inversely proportional to the elapsed time between an event and the fall (injury) (Squire, Kandel, 2009). In fact, the memory is not fixed at the moment of learning, but requires a considerable amount of time to grow into its permanent form. The consolidation process requires several steps, one of which is dependent on the medial temporal lobe structures. For as long as the process is still ongoing, the memory remains vulnerable to disintegration. Many stages of the process are completed during the first hours after learning, while the process of the memory's consolidation extends well beyond this time and involves constant changes at the level of the organization of the same long-term memory (Squire, 1987, 2004, 2007).

These results do not apply only to memory of objects or of facts, but also to autobiographical memory of events that occurred in the past. Both patients with injuries to the hippocampus and those with broader injuries to the medial temporal lobe are able to recall with precision episodes from their personal life that happened many years prior.

Squire and other scholars (2006) hypothesize that autobiographical memory of the distant past, [25] even when it involves memories full of detail and specific information about times and places, resides in the neocortex and does not involve the medial temporal lobe, in a series of studies it has been possible to demonstrate that the autobiographical memory is impaired in patients with lesions in the medial temporal cortex and prefrontal cortex. "The hippocampus seems to be essential for only a limited period of time, a period that can range from days to years depending on the species and what is being remembered. As time passes after learning, memory is reorganized and stabilized. During this period of reorganization, the role of the hippocampus gradually diminishes, and a more permanent memory is established, presumably in other cortical areas, that is independent of the hippocampal formation. One interesting idea is that the fixation process allows these other cortical areas to change gradually, slowly incorporating into their representations facts about the world and other regularities of the environment" (Squire, Kandel, 2009, p. 114). According to these considerations, therefore, the memory is probably not literally transferred from the hippocampus to the *neocortex;* rather, it is likely that there are gradual changes in the latter (including the formation of new synapses) that increase both the complexity and distribution of the mnemonic storage as well as the connections between the different cortical regions (Squire, Bayley, 2007; Squire, Kandel, 2009).

Nevertheless, Squire and Kandel have stated several times that the neuronal events on which the gradual consolidation process is based are still not well understood. In any case, as we shall see in the next paragraph, the first stage of this process takes place surely within the hippocampus itself. It is believed in fact that ultimately, long-term memory is stabilized by the accretion of the synapses that connect cortical areas to each other (Kandel, 1999; 2012).

As we showed previously, Tulving was using the term "semantic memory" to describe this type of declarative memory for organized knowledge of the world. Semantic memory can be contrasted to episodic memory, which corresponds to autobiographical memory for events that have occurred in the life of an individual. Unlike semantic memory, episodic memory stores spatial and temporal reference points, which identify the particular period and the specific place where a certain event occurred (Tulving, 1972). It is believed that semantic knowledge accumulates in cortical storage sites simply as a result of experience and thanks to the support provided by the medial temporal lobe (Squire, 1992). Instead, episodic memory seems to be based on cooperation between these cortical areas that, together with the medial temporal lobe and frontal lobes, work together to store when and where a particular event occurred. The role frontal lobes play in episodic memory becomes clear when considering up-close the nature of this type of memory, as it has an interesting implication for the nature of learning and of memory. Monkeys, rats and other living organisms are clearly able to learn and remember many things. These living systems, for example, can recall "facts," such as the fact that the choice of the red object will lead to a food reward. Until proven otherwise,[26] however, it does not appear that these animals have the capacity of episodic memory, namely to remember the moment that their choice of the red object led to getting a reward. Therefore, it seems that man alone is able to express the memory of past events in the form of "conscious autobiographical recollection of past events" (Squire, 1992). It is also possible that animals (including rats and monkeys) can express much of their memory only through actual knowledge available at the time.

In the next chapters, we will study this issue with greater care, but for now we simply highlight the fact that such a difference between man and animals would certainly make sense in terms of brain organization. One of the most obvious differences between the human and animal brain, in fact, relates to the increased size and complexity of the human associative cortex, including the regions of the frontal lobes. The frontal cortex, according to Squire and Kandel (2009), exerts a control "from top to bottom," which directs the neural activity of the sensory cortex towards the relevant sensory information. The fixing of the unique features of a particular event would be thus defined by this influence "from above," when it crosses through all the areas of the sensory cortex anatomically connected to the frontal cortex.

It was Damasio (1994, 1999, 2003), in particular, in the course of his thirty years of research on the physiology of emotions and on Alzheimer's, who suggested that many memories function in virtue of the "top to bottom" activities of higher centers that induce the cortical areas upstream to evoke specific characteristics in an image or idea. Specifically, in his 2010 volume entitled: *Self Comes to Mind. Constructing the Conscious Brain,* the great neuroscientist offers an updated version of the CDZ model,[27] a model of neural architecture he designed in the early 1990s in order to explain the processes of recollection and recognition.[28] The main part of the conceptual framework is a neural architecture of cortical connections with converging and diverging signaling properties with respect to particular nodes, called "convergence/divergence zones" (CDZ) that record the *coincidence* of the activity in neurons in different brain sites, neurons that have been activated, for example, by mapping a particular object. To be stored in memory, no part of the overall map of the object must be permanently re-represented in the CDZ: there must, instead, be registered only the coincidence of signals from the neurons associated with the map. To reconstruct the original map and thus effect the recall, Damasio suggests the mechanism of *retroactivation with synchronization.* The term *retroactivation* indicates that the mechanism needs a «return» to induce the activity; the term *synchronization* draws attention to another requirement—the need to retro-activate the components of the map in the same time span, so that what takes place simultaneously (or almost) in perception can be represented simultaneously (or almost) in the recollection. Another essential element of the conceptual framework is to postulate a division of labor between two types of brain systems: one that handles maps/images and another that regulates guidelines.

Image space, according to the great neuroscientist, is the place where the explicit images of all the sensory modes are formed: both those that become conscious, as well as those that remain unconscious. Image space is located in the enormous brain territory that creates the maps, formed by the aggregation of all the lower order sensory cortices: cortical regions located within, or near, the point where signals of a visual, auditory and other nature come to the brain. It also includes the territories of the nucleus of the solitary tract, the parabrachial nucleus and the nucleus of the upper collicoli, which have the ability to form images.

The *provision space* is, in agreement with Damasio, the place where these provisions hold both the bases of knowledge, and the dispositions for their reconstruction in the recall process. It is the source of the images in the process of imagination and reasoning, and is also used to generate movement. It is located in the cerebral cortices not otherwise occupied by image space (higher order cortices and part of the limbic cortices) and in numerous subcortical nuclei. When activated, the dispositional circuits send signals to other systems by inducing the production of images or actions (Damasio, 2007).

> The contents exhibited in the image space are *explicit,* while the contents of the dispositional space are *implicit.* We can access the contents of images, if we are conscious, but we never access the contents of dispositions directly. Of necessity, *the contents of dispositions are always unconscious.* They exist in encrypted and dormant form. Dispositions produce a variety of results. At a basic level, they can generate actions of many kinds and many levels of complexity—the release of a hormone into the bloodstream; the contraction of muscles in viscera or of muscles in a limb or in the vocal apparatus. But cortical dispositions also hold records of an image that was actually perceived on some previous occasion, and they participate in the attempt to reconstruct a sketch of that image from memory. Dispositions also assist with the processing of a currently perceived image, for instance, by influencing the degree of attention accorded to the current image (Damasio, 2010, p. 112).

In agreement with Kandel and Squire, therefore, Damasio, too, argues that all our memories—those inherited from evolution and thus available already at birth, and those acquired thereafter, thanks to learning—are in our brain in the form of provisions, waiting to become explicit images or actions. The basis of our knowledge, therefore, is implicit, encrypted and unconscious: "Dispositions are not words; they are abstract records of potentialities. The basis for the enactment of words or signs also exists as dispositions before they come to life in the form of images and actions, as in the production of speech or sign language. The rules with which we put words and signs together, the grammar of a language, are also held as dispositions" (p. 113). A convergence/divergence zone (CDZ) is a group of neurons within which many *feedforward* and *feedback* circuits come into contact. A CDZ receives feedforward connections from the sensory areas located in the "lower" level in the signal processing chain, which begin at the point where the sensory afferents enter the cerebral cortex. In turn, the CDZ sends feedback projections to those same source areas. A CDZ also sends feedforward projections towards regions that, in the chain, are located at the next connection, receiving from them return projections. The CDZ are microscopic and are located within the convergence/divergence regions (CDR), which instead are macroscopic. Damasio believes the number of CDZs to be in the tens of thousands, and the number of CDRs to be in the dozens. The CDZs are micronodes; CDRs are macronodes. The CDR are located, within the associative cortices, in strategic areas where several fundamental pathways converge (Damasio, 1989, 1994, 2003, 2010).

Thanks to studies of experimental neuroanatomy, we know that such connectivity configurations exist in the brains of non-human primates (Rockland, Pandya, 1979). In addition, we are aware, based on recent neuro-imaging studies conducted with magnetic resonance using various diffusion techniques, of the fact that such configurations exist also in human beings (Hagmann *et al.*, 2008). As we will see later, the CDR are important in the production and organization of the essential content of the conscious mind, including those that compose the self. Both the CDR and the CDZ come into being under genetic control. When the body interacts with the environment during development, synaptic strengthening or weakening introduces significant changes in the convergence regions and brings about maximal change in the CDZs. Synaptic strengthening takes place when the outside conditions correspond to the body's survival needs (Damasio, 2010).[29]

In light of all this, therefore, the task that Damasio imagines for the CDZ is to recreate separate configurations of neural activity that during perception had occurred in roughly a simultaneous manner, i.e. occurring in the same time window necessary for us to become aware of and pay attention to them. To achieve this, the CDZ will cause a very rapid activation sequence—not detected by consciousness—that will bring separate neural regions to "connect" in a certain order. The great neuroscientist writes: "In this architecture, knowledge retrieval would be based on relatively simultaneous, attended activity in many early cortical regions, engendered over several reiterations of such reactivation cycles. Those separate activities would be the basis of reconstructed representations. The level at which knowledge is retrieved would depend on the scope of multiregional activation. In turn, this would depend on the level of CDZ that is activated" (p. 116).

Damasio and Meyer recently analyzed a large number of studies in the field of perception, imagination and "mirror" processing by interpreting the results from the perspective of the convergence/divergence model (Meyer, Damasio, 2009): many of them seem to be interesting verifications of the model in question. Specifically, data from both functional neuro-imaging research and from studies of injuries indicates that, in the cortex, the recollection of objects and events relies at least in part on activity taking place at both the sensory afferents' input areas and at the motor efferents' output areas (Kiefer *et al.*, 2008; Hagen *et al.*, 2002). Naturally, it is no coincidence that these are the same sites engaged in the original perception of objects and events. Moreover, research on mirror neurons, to which topic a part of the last chapter of this book is dedicated, is providing evidence that an architecture based on convergence/divergence offers a satisfactory explanation of some complex phenomena (mental operations and behaviors). As we will see later, the research into mirror neurons has provided the key result that the mere observation of an action is sufficient to activate the corresponding motor areas in the brain (Rizzolatti, Craighero, 2004); this last observation could be easily explained with the CDZ model (Damasio, Meyer, 2008).

Although the model presented here provides a very reliable explanation of the processes of recall and recognition, the understanding of these complex dynamics is not complete, unless accompanied by a detailed knowledge of the molecular mechanisms that underlie declarative memory storage in the long term. So far we have shown how both types of memory (explicit and implicit) are deposited in the respective sensory and motor systems that initially processed the information. However, while the learning of a non-declarative memory directly regulates the efficiency of the neurons in these areas, the storage of long-term declarative memory requires an additional neural loop, i.e., an additional system, namely, the hippocampus and other medial temporal lobe structures. Since declarative memory requires conscious remembering, we can therefore ask whether this type of memory also requires a series of particular synaptic and molecular mechanisms. We will address these issues in the next paragraph.

2.5 Long-term potentiation and the consolidation switch

According to the idea that the role of the hippocampus and other parts of the medial temporal lobe is one of modulating the initial representation formed in cortical areas when information is processed for the first time, we can see how hippocampus plays a linking function. To connect the storage sites, found independently in numerous cortical regions (Squire, Kandel, 2009).

In 1973 T. Bliss and T. Lomo found that repeated synaptic activation induces a lasting increase in the effectiveness of excitatory synaptic transmission in the hippocampus. Aware of Milner's results, the two Norwegian scholars stimulated specific nerve pathways in a rabbit's hippocampus, demonstrating that neural activity influences synaptic strength (Bliss, Lomo, 1973). Today we know that this type of facilitation is part of a family of processes rather than a single process, with each stage based on a series of slightly different second messengers (Squire, Bayley, 2007). Some of these second messenger molecules act in postsynaptic center, while others carry out their action in the presynaptic neuron and others on both sides of the synapse. This set of processes is commonly referred to as *long-term potentiation* (LTP) and consists in the long-term facilitation of communication between two neurons, as a result of the prolonged activation of the synapse that connects them (Bliss *et al.*, 2004; Posner *et al.*, 2009). Many features of the LTP make this phenomenon the most plausible biological substrate for memory formation and for the codification of the brain changes induced by experience.

Firstly, the LTP occurs within each of the two main pathways that lead information to the hippocampus, namely the temporo-direct ammonia, which leads from the entorhinal cortex to the pyramidal cells of the CA1 region, and each of the three components of the indirect pathway: the perforating pathway, the pathway of the mucous fibers and the Schaffer collateral pathway. Secondly, LTP is induced quickly: a single download of high-frequency electrical stimulation can double the strength of the synaptic connection. Thirdly, once induced, LTP is stable for one or more hours or even days, depending on the number of times that the tetanus is repeated. In a manner similar to long-term facilitation in *Aplysia,* we mentioned above, LTP therefore possesses the characteristics of the mnemonic process itself: i.e., it can be induced quickly at certain synapses and be long lasting (Nicoll *et al.*, 1988).

The mere fact, however, that LTP has features in common with an ideal storage process does not prove that this is the exact mechanism used by cells to store memory. However, and this is Kandel and Squire's belief, if we could prove that LTP carries out a causative role in memory, then the scientific community would find itself before a great opportunity to study the storage mechanisms of a kind of memory that is very difficult to analyze under normal conditions. The LTP, therefore, has the advantage of being produced in the laboratory, that is, under controlled conditions, which make it easier to identify the molecular mechanisms underlying mnemonic processes (Wang *et al.*, 2005). Though LTP can be induced in numerous synapses of the hippocampus and in many regions of the cerebral cortex, the mechanisms responsible for its induction are not always the same. In fact, these mechanisms vary not only within the various synapses but also, in some cases, within a single synapse. This happens, for example, when different stimulation frequencies or patterns are applied to induce facilitation. Detailed studies indicate that these mechanisms may be of at least two main types: associative and nonassociative (Kandel *et. al.*, 2000).

In *Aplysia*, the dentate gyrus receives information from the entorhinal cortex and conveys this information to the hippocampus through grainy cells. From these, emanate axons in a bundle of fibers, called the *pathway of the mucous fibers,* which terminate in the pyramidal neurons of the CA3 region of the hippocampus. The mucous membranes use the neurotransmitter glutamate. In the fiber mucous, the LTP has some features in common with the facilitation of the *Aplysia* neurons during sensitization. In fact, in a manner similar to long-term facilitation that contributes to sensitization, the LTP of mucous membranes is non-associative (Kandel, 1983a, 1983b). It does not depend on postsynaptic activity or on other signals reaching these membranes at the same time. This form of LTP is caused simply by a short train of high-frequency neuronal activity in the presynaptic neurons and by the consequent influx of calcium ions. Within the presynaptic neuron, the calcium ions, in turn, induce a series of familiar stages. In particular, these ions activate a calcium-calmodulin-dependent cyclase adenylate (type I); this enzyme acts in such a way as to increase the level of cAMP, which in turn activates cAMP-dependent protein kinase (PKA). As we saw earlier, "the cAMP-dependent protein kinase adds phosphate groups to proteins and thereby activates some proteins and inhibits others" (Squire, Kandel, 2009, p. 125). Although the precise role played by LTP of mucous membranes in memory is still unclear, a better correlation between declarative memory and LTP is observed in other hippocampal pathways: the Schaffer collateral pathway and the direct temporo ammonic pathway (Squire, 2007).

Schaffer collateral pathways are formed by the pyramidal cells of the hippocampal CA3 region sending axons to CA1 region cells. The synaptic endings of the Schaffer collateral pathways also release the glutamate neurotransmitter, but, unlike the mucous membranes, in the Schaffer collateral pathway LTP is induced only when the postsynaptic cell triggers the NMDA (the N- methyl-D- Aspartase receptor) receptor that binds the glutamate (Harvey, Svoboda, 2007). Therefore, this form of LTP is associative; it requires the concomitant activity of both the pre- and postsynaptic cell. Thanks to a series of complex experiments, Wigström and Gustaffson (1988) applied the properties of the NMDA receptor to the context of LTP. Demonstrating that LTP did not require only the sending of pulses by the presynaptic neuron, but that these trains of pulses also had to be repeated in order to substantially depolarize the postsynaptic neurons and therefore remove the cap of Mg^{2+} ions from the opening of the canal of the NMDA receptor. According to these scholars, only in this case would the amount of Ca^{2+} ions, which entered the cell through the NMDA receptor channels, be enough to initiate the series of stages leading to a persistent increase in synaptic transmission. "This finding as it provided the first direct evidence for Hebb's proposal, which stated that 'when an axon of cell A [. . .] excites cell B and repeatedly or persistently takes part in firing it, some growth process or metabolic change takes place in one or both cells so that A's efficiency as one of the cells firing B is increased.' Synapses that exhibit this property are now called Hebb synapses" (Squire, Kandel, 2009, p. 127). The kick that penetrates the postsynaptic cell triggers at least three different protein kinases: the calcium-calmodulin-dependent protein kinase II (CaM Kinase II), protein kinase C and a tyrosine kinase (fyn). Although all three of these kinases differ from the cAMP-dependent protein kinase we mentioned in the previous paragraphs, they seem to have a similar function: these kinases carry out phosphorylation by adding phosphate groups to specific target proteins, thereby activating certain proteins and inhibiting others (Squire, Kandel, 2009). So far we have mentioned that LTP is a phenomenon that can be produced in the laboratory in a completely artificial manner. We cannot therefore assume that it necessarily reflects what happens during the storage of memory. At this point in the examination, then, we may wonder if memory storage makes use of LTP, and, if so, we may wonder what is its role. Here we'll look at the first issue, once more by following in the direction of Kandel and Squire's research approach (Kandel, Squire, 2000) who verified "If LTP is a mechanism for memory storage in the hippocampus, then defects in LTP should interfere with the declarative memory. In the rat, as in humans, lesions of the hippocampus interfere with the formation of new spatial memories, that is, memory for places, which is a form of declarative memory" (Squire, Kandel, 2009, p. 130). Is it possible, for instance, to disactivate LTP and continue to store spatial memories?

The use of inhibitors to analyze a behavior or a biochemical pathway poses a problem, because often the inhibitors are not entirely specific. These substances can, for example, block other receptors as well, or can act on other molecules and the effect observed could, plausibly, be a result of this latter action. In this regard, in 1990 research on memory made great progress thanks to the development of the methodology of knock-out genes. This technique allows you to manipulate any gene of the mice genome and has therefore made it possible to analyze the way in which a single gene acts on both LTP and memory (Mayford *et al.*, 1996).

Capecchi (1990) and Smithies (Reid *et al.*, 1991) have offered a substantial contribution in developing the technique of targeted gene ablation in the stem cells of mouse embryos, devising an excellent genetic system to relate individual genes to synaptic plasticity, on the one hand, and the more complex forms of declarative memory, on the other.[30] The medial temporal lobe of mice, hippocampus included, is reminiscent of that of humans, and in these animals, too, the hippocampus is involved in storing locations and objects. Although we do not yet know much about how the information is processed in the hippocampus, it has by now been ascertained that it contains a cellular representation of extrapersonal space—a cognitive map of this space—and that lesions to this area interfere with spatial tasks. In 1992, in fact, Kandel and colleagues applied the knock-out techniques to the study of LTP and learning in mice, demonstrating that animals lack one of the two genes that encode kinases of second messengers showed a reduced LTP (Grant *et al.*, 1992). Since the deletion of these genes did not interfere in any observable way with the normal behavior of these mice, it was therefore possible to study their learning and recall abilities. Thus it was seen that the interference with the two kinases had effects on spatial memory: animals continued to get lost in the maze even after many learning trials. Regardless of the degree of manipulation, the gene knock-out technique poses a potential problem: since the induced defect is present from the earliest stages of life the mice could be subject to abnormal development. In this sense, the lack of LTP and spatial memory may actually be the result of some developmental problems, such as the formation of abnormal connections in the Schaffer collateral pathway. This possibility was reduced through the use of a second type of mutant mouse in which a transgene could be turned on and off by giving it a specific drug. In this second type of mouse, a mutated form of calcium-calmodulin-dependent kinase–one of the three kinases essential for LTP- was overexpressed throughout the hippocampus. Overexpression caused an interference with LTP and a defect in spatial memory. However, when the transgene was turned off, LTP became normal and the animal's memory capability was restored. These experiments strengthen the correlation between some aspects of LTP within the CA1 pyramidal neurons of the hippocampus and spatial memory (Squire, Kandel, 2009). These results raise another question: why does the interference with LTP negatively affect spatial memory storage? How does LTP induce the depositing of these memories?

Frey, Huang, Nguyen and Kandel tried to determine whether LTP was influenced by the repetition of the stimulus (Frey *et al.*, 1993; Nguyen *et al.*, 1994), finding that the hippocampal LTP proceeds in stages, similar to the way facilitation occurs in *Aplysia.* The early phase of LTP, produced by a single train of stimuli, only lasts few hours and does not require new protein synthesis (Nguyen *et al.*, 1994); it provides covalent modifications of pre-existing proteins that strengthen existing connections, similar to what happens in the short term facilitation in *Aplysia.*[31] Instead, repeated trains of electrical stimuli produce the late stage of LTP, which has quite different properties compared to early LTP, and is more similar to long-term facilitation in *Aplysia.* The late phase of LTP persists for at least a day and requires both the processes of translation and transcription. Just like implicit long-term memory, the late phase of LTP requires PKA, MAPK and CREB, and results in the development of new synaptic connections (Bolshakov *et al.*, 1997; Bourtchouladze *et al.*, 1994; Engert, Bonhoeffer, 1999; Frey *et al.*, 1993; Nguyen *et al.*, 1994)[32]. These mechanisms also play a role in the visual cortex where it is believed that they take part in the regulation of synaptic connections during advanced stages of normal development. Therefore, despite the logical and anatomical differences that distinguish declarative memory from non-declarative, the basic mechanisms of long-term storage in these two types of memory have some common traits.

To investigate further the specific role of PKA and late LTP in memory, Abel, Kandel and others scholars have created transgenic mice that express R (AB), a mutant form of the regulatory subunit of PKA that inhibits the activity of the enzyme (Abel *et al.*, 1997). The reduction of PKA activity in the hippocampus is accompanied by a significant decrease in late LTP reflecting in problems of long-term memory functioning linked to the hippocampus regarding extrapersonal space, while learning and short-term memory remain intact. Then, in the explicit memory of extrapersonal space, linked to the hippocampus of mammals, PKA plays a key role in the conversion of short-term memory into long-term memory, similar to what happens in the implicit memory of *Aplysia* and *Drosophila*. As a result of what was observed in R(A/B) mice, Kandel and colleagues wondered why animals with deficiencies in their PKA signaling system encountered difficulties of a spatial nature (Abel *et al.*, 1997). In doing so, scholars drew inspiration from the famous research case done by O'Keefe and Dostrovsky, to whom we owe the discovery, in 1971, that hippocampal pyramidal cells—which, in the LTP studies, are examined by electrically stimulating the Shaffer collateral pathway—are place cells that allow the animal to encode extrapersonal space (O'Keefe, Nadel, 1978). A pyramidal cell will fire only when the mouse's head is in a certain position in a circumscribed area of space. If it is placed in a new environment, in a few minutes the animal develops an internal representation of the space (thanks to firing activity coordinated by a population of place cells), which usually remains stable for days. If it is placed in a second environment, it builds a new map due in part to some cells that made up the first environment and partly to pyramidal cells that had previously been inactive (O'Keefe, Nadel, 1978). This spatial map constitutes researchers' best-understood example of a complex internal representation of the brain, a real cognitive map. This configuration differs in several ways from the classic sensory maps identified, for example, in visual systems. Unlike sensory maps, in fact, the spatial map is not of a topographic type, i.e. adjacent cells of the hippocampus do not represent adjacent regions in the environment. The place cells' activity, in fact, may persist even when the relevant sensory stimuli have been removed or when the animal is in a dark environment (Squire, 1987, 2004). Therefore, it seems that the place cells do not create a map of the actual sensory input, but that they form a picture of the place where the animal is believed to be (Squire, Kandel, 2009).[33]

In such circumstances, therefore, according to Kandel (2012) we can infer that such experiments provide the first link in the causal chain for generating declarative memory, which, at the level of man, binds the molecules to the mind, since it illustrates the way in which genes affect the connections between cells and how these changes affect, in turn, an internal representation that guides a complex behavior of the living system. Specifically, interference with the LTP of hippocampal CA1 pyramidal cells also influences the normal operation of spatial fields—the internal representation of space. Deficiencies in LTP cause alterations over time, in particular, in the stability of the spatial maps that, in turn, reveal themselves in the form of unstable spatial memory (Serulle *et al.*, 2007; Wang *et al.*, 2005).

One aspect that struck Kandel from the beginning of his research was, therefore, the close similarity between learning processes and the formation of new maps. The map develops as the animal becomes familiar with the surrounding space and, once learned, it persists for days or even weeks. In a first study, designed to test whether the molecular mechanisms sustaining late-phase LTP had a role in the long-term stabilization of this configuration, Kentros, Muller, Hawkins and Kandel limited themselves to blocking LTP pharmaceutically with an antagonist of the NMDA receptor (Kentros *et al.*, 1998). If placed in a new environment, the animal is able to create a proper map of the surrounding area that remains stable after an hour. Most pyramidal cells do not retain the representation of a previously acquired field for more than 24 hours. This makes us think that activation of the NMDA receptors—which perhaps represents an important step in the process of synaptic efficacy changes—is required for long-term stabilization of the map of place cells, a result consistent with the role of the late phase of LTP in this consolidation process. Kandel and colleagues therefore wondered whether a selective impairment that affects only the late phase of LTP may cause a selective anomaly in the long-term stability of the cells. Since only the late phase of LTP requires PKA, Rotenberg, Muller, Abel, Hawkins and Kandel again used transgenic R(AB) mice with a decrease of PKA activity and a reduced form of late LTP (Rotenberg *et al.*, 2000). While it is true that the reduced PKA activity influences the stability of the place cells, then the R(A/B) mice should be able to create a stable map of the space in a new environment, like normal animals, which lasts for at least one hour; the range of the same cell should instead become unstable after twenty-four hours. This theory was confirmed by observations made by Kandel and colleagues. The similarities found between the long-term instability of the spatial map, memory deficits in the long term and the deficits of the late stage of LTP suggest that gene activation mediated by PKA and the synthesis of new proteins could have an essential role in the stabilization of the map of the surrounding space. Agnihotri, Kentros Hawkins and Kandel have submitted this hypothesis to verification, discovering that, by inhibiting protein synthesis, one destabilizes the position fields in the long term, more or less as occurs with PKA inhibition (Kentros *et al.*, 2001; Kandel, 2001).[34]

What emerged from a study by Kandel and colleagues and another study was that the balance between protein phosphorylation regulated by PKA and dephosphorylation determine the threshold of the hippocampus's synaptic plasticity and memory (Malleret *et al.*, 2001). To determine whether the Ca^{2+}-dependent endogenous phosphatase acts as an inhibitory regulator of this balance, Kandel and colleagues blocked the action by examining the effects of the intervention on the synaptic plasticity of the mouse's memory. Later studies have found that transient reduction of calcineurin activity causes a facilitation of LTP both *in vitro* and *in vivo* which persists for several days in the whole (intact) animal and is accompanied by improved learning and by a consolidation of the memory in the short and long term in several spatial and non-spatial tasks involving the hippocampus (Malleret et al. 2001). These findings, reveal that overexpression of calcineurin inhibits the PKA-dependent components of LTP and memory and thus show that endogenous calcineurin can act as a negative regulator in synaptic plasticity, learning and memory (Mansuy et al. 1998; Kandel, 2001).[35]

In light of all this, therefore, the studies by Kandel and his colleagues on the storage component of memories have led to two general conclusions. In first place, the research suggests that cellular and molecular strategies employed by *Aplysia* in the storage of information in short-term memory and long-term are preserved with evolution and are also used in the implicit and explicit memory faculty in mammals. In both forms of memory, various stages can be seen associated with changes in synaptic efficacy and that are related to behavioral stages of memory in the short and long term. The synaptic changes in the short term involve covalent modification of preexisting proteins, which in turn reflect modifications of pre-existing synaptic connections, while long-term changes involve the activation of gene expression, the synthesis of new proteins and the formation of new connections. However, while the short-term deposit of implicit and explicit memories requires different signals, the long-term memory of both implicit and explicit memories employs a major signaling pathway linked to the combined action of PKA, MAPK and CREB-1. At least in mice, it is likely that there are more mechanisms at play. Both in explicit and implicit memory, the transition from short-term to form long-term is regulated by inhibitory controls. In the second place, research on learning has shown new aspects of synaptic transmission and new histological features related to synaptic signaling activity. The different forms of learning have different neurotransmitter modulators, which can act in three ways: a) activate second messenger kinases, which are transported into the nucleus and there initiate processes necessary for the growth of neurons and for long-term memory; b) mark specific synapses, making them susceptible to the process in the long-term and adjusting the *in situ* protein synthesis necessary for stabilization; c) mediate, in ways that we only now are beginning to understand, the attention processes necessary for the formation and evocation of memory. One aspect worth mentioning is that the study of long-term memory has enabled us to understand the existence of a close dialogue between the synapses and the nucleus, and vice versa (Squire, Kandel, 2009). In the long-term process, a synapse's response is not only determined by its antecedent activity (as in short-term plasticity) but also by the activation of the process of transcription in the nucleus. We began this chapter by pointing out how Kandel believed that a reductionist approach based on the use of a simple experimental setup (e.g. *Aplysia*) would allow us to address fundamental issues such as learning and memory.

However, Kandel in many of his more recent articles does not negate the considerable complexity of declarative memory, a type of memory, that is, which in some regards is still little known (Kandel, 2001, 2009, 2012; Squire, Kandel, 2009). To wit, still to be explored are several molecular mechanisms that induce or stabilize synaptic growth associated with long-term memory. So far, only the molecular mechanisms of memory function have been examined. The most complex aspect of memory—and specifically, that of declarative memory—involves its systemic organization. Many are the important questions at this level that remain unanswered. How, for example, do the different regions of the hippocampus and medial temporal lobe—the subicular, entorhinal, parahippocampal and perineal areas—interact when information for explicit memory is deposited? How is information transferred from these regions to the neocortex, where it is consolidated definitively? Neither do we know, for that matter, why the hippocampus is involved in the initial depositing of information in the long-term memory, while it is much less involved once the memory has been stored for weeks or months (Milner *et al.*, 1998; Squire, Zola-Morgan, 199; Kandel, 2001). Which essential information is transmitted from the hippocampus to the neocortex? Lastly, we know almost nothing about the nature of the process of recalling memories contained in explicit (declarative) memory, a process that requires conscious activity. These problems of a systemic nature, which we will address in the following chapters, will require integrating the *bottom-up* approach used by molecular biology, with the *top-down* approach of cognitive science, complexity science and psychiatry, as well as, more generally, the philosophy of mind and the bioeducative sciences. In other words, what will be needed is a theoretical synthesis capable of holding together methodological reductionism, on the one hand, and holism on the other. Despite all its complexity, in fact, the question, with many of its implications, concerning the mystery of the self that comes to mind in a conscious brain capable of discovering, creating, transmitting and assimilating ever new meanings, in these last few years, has arisen in new ways thanks to surprising and counter-intuitive discoveries (Damasio, 2010). Besides Kandel and Squire, among the living experts there are Damasio, Siegel, Searle, Edelman and Freeman who, while moving from positions in some cases quite different from each other, in any rate find themselves in accord in taking up an anti-dualistic perspective. One can think, in that sense, of the relationship between archaic brain regions, such as the amygdala, and the more recent regions, like the prefrontal cortex, in the genesis of moral choices and decision-making processes. These antidualistic foundations are then integrated by new and complex sequences: that of the influence of primal emotions and feelings (pleasure and pain) as connective bridges between the proto-self and the self; that of the distinction between brain states and mental states, together with the memory in the construction of individual identity; as well as those concerning the close relationship that exists between biological information, intentionality, self-organization and cognition in the comparison between humans and other animals (starting with primates) or differences between the vegetative state and the forms of minimal consciousness in the infinite range of perceptual and cognitive nuances. As we shall see, one of the results of this multi-faceted exploration will be the idea of consciousness and memory as natural processes,[36] an authentic way of avoiding both dualism and monism which utilizes and masterfully brings to fruition a brilliant intuition of W. James.

Chapter 3

Self-consciousness and Causality

3.1 The "nature"of consciousness and neurobiological explorations

As we saw in the previous chapter, the work of Kandel and his colleagues today has given us a real code capable of allowing molecular biology and cognitive science to communicate. It is a synthesis that sheds new light on human complexity and in particular on the mysteries of consciousness and memory (Squire, Kandel, 2009). In a nutshell, we can infer that there are at least four fundamental discoveries of the Austrian psychiatrist. Firstly, the mechanisms of memory consist in changes in synaptic transmission and are conserved between species. These modifications can occur at both the pre- and post-synaptic level and, above all, synapses of the same type can be modified in different ways and also opposed to the various types of learning. Secondly, in addition to synaptic transmission, learning also affects the excitability of the neurons. Therefore, even the discharge properties of a neuron are subject to modification, helping to transform the synapses and neural circuits. Thirdly, the synaptic modifications induced by learning may involve different temporal stages, contributing to the forms of short-term and long-term memory; hierarchical and stratified, but not necessarily identical, cellular processes contribute to the different temporal stages. Fourthly, the changes concerning memory do not only affect synaptic functioning but also promote structural changes in the synaptic contacts. The short-term storage of information involves covalent modifications of pre-existing proteins, whereas long-term memory requires changes in gene expression and, thus, the synthesis of new proteins (Kandel, 2001, 2012).

However, to fully understand the functioning of the biological substrates of cognitive processes, it is necessary, in line with Kandel's research, to go beyond the study of individual neurons and analyze the ways in which neural networks process information. The Austrian scholar has shown that we readily acquire and retain new information because the brain systems important for memory are quickly modified. The synaptic connections in these systems can be strengthened or weakened and are even capable of permanent structural changes. This remarkable plasticity of the brain constitutes, for Kandel, the biological basis of individuality and all aspects of mental life. To explore these issues in depth, however, one should not only consider the methods and approaches that the neurosciences use to study cells and neural systems, but also draw on the analytical potential of the cognitive sciences. Substantial evidence of the profound influence that experience exerts on the brain has been derived from studies on perception, that is, the way we interpret the information coming from the world, by giving it a meaning. We experience external reality through our senses. Each feeling is first analyzed by the respective receptors located at the body's surface and then forwarded to the cerebral cortex, passing through special nerve centers.

Current research on the role of the cerebral cortex in sensation owes much to the pioneering studies carried out by Marshall, Woolsey and Bard (1937), who discovered that the body surface of monkeys was represented on the surface of their brains, in the form of a sensory map. The cortical neurons are neatly grouped in such a way as to form a map of the body. Adjacent skin areas terminate and are represented in adjacent areas of the cortex. The neurosurgeon Penfield (1952, 1958) subsequently confirmed the existence of a similar sensory map in humans, demonstrating that there is a naked representation of the body not only monkeys' brains, but in those of humans as well. The cortical representation of the human body is like a person—a homunculus—whose right side of the body is represented in the left hemisphere and vice versa (Penfield, Rasmussen, 1952). Until not long ago, it was thought that this cortical representation remained unchanged from one individual to another and did not undergo changes in an individual's lifetime.

This idea was refuted by experiments carried out by Merzenich and colleagues, who found that cerebral representations varied significantly from one monkey to another (Merzenich, Sameshine, 1993). These observations were also confirmed by subsequent experiments conducted by the same group. These studies show that the cortical maps of the body's surface are not static, but dynamic. They are constantly revised with the use over time of the sensory pathways. The functional connections may therefore increase or decrease depending on usage. Since each of us experiences different sensory and social environments and because no two people experience exactly the same environment, over the course of each person's lifetime their brain is changed in different ways. This gradual generation of an exclusive brain architecture constitutes, in Kandel's eyes, the biological condition for the emergence of individuality (Kandel, Squire, 2000; Squire, Kandel, 2009). With regard to the tactile sense, the mechanism appears to be similar to that used for associative long-term potentiation (LTP) in the hippocampus. In the cortical map, the areas simultaneously active on the skin tend to be shown together. Merzenich and colleagues illustrated this principle by surgically joining the skin of the third and fourth finger of a hand. The two fingers were, therefore, always used together and the information coming from the skin of these fingers was constantly correlated, as in the case of associative LTP. The surgery had changed in an evident manner the cerebral representation of the cortical area corresponding to the hand. In fact, the precise boundaries that normally separate the areas corresponding to the third and fourth finger had disappeared. Therefore, although the area corresponding to the cortical representation of each finger is usually precisely bounded, the configuration and size of these connections can be modified by experience, by simply changing the time frame of the information coming from the fingers (Squire, Kandel, 2009).

In these circumstances, therefore, research on touch and its cortical representation at the level of the anterior areas of the parietal lobe provide simple examples of the internal representation of the body surface and of the peripersonal space. The analysis of the modifications of this representation at the level of the posterior parietal association cortex indicates that attention processes entail the integration of the internal representation of the body with vision and movement, which causes the representation of the personal space to be further integrated with the representation of the extrapersonal space (Kandel, 2001; Albright *et al.*, 2000). In this way, the representation of the body is related to both the representation of visual space and with the image and memory we have of it, and it is precisely within this integrated representation that self-consciousness operates (Kandel *et al.*, 2000). Therefore, it is perhaps unsurprising that the Russian neuropsychologist Luria (1980) hypothesized that at the level of certain regions of the parietal lobe, we may find the most distinctly human characteristics of cortical organization. The neurons of the primary somatosensory cortex project to the higher order association areas of the anterior parietal cortex and to the multimodal associative areas of the posterior parietal cortex (Brodmann areas 5 and 7).

The association areas of the posterior parietal cortex also receive afferent connections from the visual and auditory systems and from the hippocampus. Therefore, these associative areas integrate the somatosensory information with that of other sensory modalities and this integration is a fundamental process for perceiving three-dimensional characteristics of objects and knowing how to manipulate them. In no cortical area are the relationships between higher mental processes and activities of the nerve cells so evident as in the posterior parietal cortex. Lesions to this area do not cause simple sensory deficits such as loss of tactile sensitivity, but agnosia. Complex disorders are associated with agnosia, such as deficits in spatial perception, visuomotor integration and selective attention. The forms of agnosia most commonly observed as a result of lesions to the right posterior parietal cortex responsible for the processing of visual information are among the most surprising forms that can be observed in patients with neurological diseases (Kandel *et al.*, 2000).

Research conducted on patients with neglect syndrome resulting from injuries to the right hemisphere showed deficiencies related to the perception of the shape of objects. These patients are not able to "see" all the parts of an object; even if their visual pathways are intact, they nevertheless fail to recognize some parts. These clinical observations have provided the first evidence that the perceptual pathways also include specific circuits responsible for examining the overall shape of the objects and particular aspects specific to that shape (Kandel et al. 2000). This means that the memory of the extrapersonal space is stored according to a reference system centered on the body. Recent surveys by the TEP have shown that when subjects are asked to close their eyes and mentally visualize the view of an object, the primary visual cortex is activated, as happens when one really looks at an object. This means that the visual images generated by the imagination are mediated by the same parts of the visual system that in turn are involved in processing images generated directly by visual stimuli (Squire, Kandel, 2009). For this reason, lesions of the posterior parietal cortex, which cause deficits in the visual perception of objects observed in real time, cause deficits also in the creation of visual images through memory and imagination. Furthermore, it has been observed that many tasks requiring one to imagine things visually by drawing on the warehouses of the memory cause an intense activation of the posterior parietal cortex, which suggests that in their imagination individuals orient their bodies with respect to the figures generated by their imagination (Kandel *et al.*, 2000). Presumably, in accordance with Kandel, it is precisely this ability to orient oneself thanks to the imagination that is lacking in patients with representational neglect.

The studies just mentioned also allow us to delve into the nature of consciousness one of the greatest mysteries of cognitive neuroscience. The peculiarities of this mysterious phenomenon arouse great interest, provoking lively debate among scientists, philosophers and theologians. In particular, it is difficult for some to accept the idea, of a materialist and reductionist stamp, that consciousness can only be explained by recourse to immanent causes of a physical-chemical nature. Kandel, in his now-famous book entitled: *Principles of Neural Science*, says that,

> what we commonly call the mind is simply the entire set of operations of the brain. In this sense, consciousness is fundamentally a function of the brain and therefore in principle we should be able to identify neural mechanisms that give rise to consciousness. This, of course, does not begin to tell us what to look for in the brain. We must first come to terms with the defining characteristics of consciousness if we are to develop productive neural theories of consciousness (Kandel *et al.*, 2000, p. 396).

These words are the very heart of this great scientist's thought. The molecular biology of cognition promises to complete the circle leading from the mind to molecules by assuming that consciousness is a biological process explainable in terms of molecular signaling pathways used by populations of nerve cells in communication with each other. Thus, according to Kandel, the brain is merely an "information-processing computational organ made marvelously powerful not by its mystery, but by its complexity—by the enormous number, variety, and interactions of its nerve cells" (Kandel, 2006, p. 10).

The new science of the mind, therefore, through a deep understanding of the biology of memory, does not limit itself to finding solutions for devastating diseases. It aims "to penetrate the mystery of consciousness, including the ultimate mystery: how each person's brain creates the consciousness of a unique self and the sense of free will" (p. 12). This conclusion serves as the reference point for each *strong* strategy of naturalization, in the sense of expressions such as that of "morality gene" or "biological ethics" (Wilson, 1980). This seems to be flanked by the advancement of knowledge regarding the continuity between *Homo sapiens* and the animal species closest to him, along the lines of the titles of the best known works of Frans de Waal, as well as recent development in neuroscience, which have paved the way for neuroethics as an explanation of moral reasoning based on the brain: the new neuroimaging techniques would provide the tool to solve once and for all the problem of translating the prescriptive (moral) content of experience into the purely descriptive terms of a chemical-physical reality (Semplici, 2009a). Yet it is precisely Gazzaniga who warns against the hypertrophic temptation of the new brain-based philosophy of life he promotes: "In spite of a growing body of research that suggests that the brain does indeed determine the mind, this does not mean that there is no such thing as personal responsibility" (Gazzaniga, 2006, p. 148).

Edelman takes up the Hegelian idea of second nature as the logical culmination of the theory of neural Darwinism, that is, the awareness that the history of the species and the individual is constructed by combining selective, adaptive and interactive processes between the body and the natural and cultural environment (Edelman, 2006). The result is an open conception of subjectivity, which manages to incorporate both the play of sentiments and the pressure of socio-cultural forces and education, with the result that a radically reductionist explanation of all of that is continuously added to the *first* nature through perceptions, categorical intuitions, memories, individual and collective attitudes, is neither "desirable nor probable or imminent" (Edelman, 1990, 2006; Semplici, 2009a). Searle, for example, has no doubt that consciousness is an ordinary biological phenomenon just like digestion, photosynthesis or the secretion of enzymes. And yet it is from these "secretions" that the reality of something like money depends, which is never simply a piece of paper or a metal disk and at some point becomes completely independent of the physical support upon which we regularly see it circulate (Searle, 1992, 2002). This complexity cuts deep into the biological evolutionary side of science. Consciousness, in fact, is not just about the images present in the mind. At the very least, it involves an organization of the contents of the mind that have their center in the same organism that produces them, and is the source of their motivation. Consciousness, on the other hand, is more than an organized mind under the influence of a living, acting organism. It is also a mind, able to know that such a living, acting organism exists. Of course, the brain's ability to create neural patterns that map objects experienced as images is an important part of the process of consciousness. The orientation of these images in the organism's internal perspective also forms part of the process (Damasio, 2010).

The mere presence of organized images that flow in a mental stream is enough to produce a mind; but if a few additional processes are not added, it remains an unconscious mind: what is missing is a self. According to Searle, to become conscious the brain must acquire a new property: subjectivity. A defining trait of subjectivity is the feeling that pervades the subjectively experienced images.

In *The Mystery of Consciousness*, Searle (1997) offers a modern treatment of the importance of subjectivity seen from the perspective of philosophy. In line with this idea, the decisive step in the creation of consciousness is not the formation of images or the creation of the basis of a mind. The decisive step lies in making the images our own, in making them belong to their rightful owners, that is, to the individual, perfectly delineated organisms in which they emerge. Subjectivity is thus the peculiar characteristic that Searle and, independently, Nagel (1995) attribute to consciousness, and is also that which generates the most debate in science. The other two are unity and intentionality.

The unitary nature of consciousness refers to the fact that we see our experiences as a unified whole. All the different sensory modalities are blended in a single conscious experience. Our perceptions, in fact, do not appear as a single unit only for the short duration of our experience, but continue to be experienced as a whole over time. When we talk to our guests, we do so with complete sentences and pay little or no attention at all to the process of constructing the sentence, although we are aware that we are formulating a concept (Kandel *et al.* 2000; Albright, 2000). Finally, consciousness has intentionality.[1] Our experiences continue to retain their meaning beyond the physical sensations of the moment in which we have them. Our mind is able to bring together and represent the whole range of our experiences. In *Intentionality* (1983) Searle develops a general theory of mental phenomena that refers to the phenomenological tradition of Brentano and Husserl, but within a realistic perspective, radically different from Brentano's psychologism and Husserl's transcendentalism. For Brentano, intentionality constitutes the peculiar characteristic of psychic phenomena and that which distinguishes them from physical phenomena.[2]

With Husserl intentionality is no longer an extensive concept, characterizing mental states in general; rather it becomes the defining trait of consciousness. "It is intentionality which characterizes consciousness in the pregnant sense," as it is "the property of the *Erlebnisse* to be conscious" (Husserl, 1952a, pp. 109–110). It becomes the basic starting point for the construction of a real cognitive method, a philosophical notion able to penetrate the world of man's consciousness.

The fundamental character of intentionality, the "direction towards an object," is a property which Searle, too, accepts, along with the trait of being irreducible to something else. Like Husserl, Searle considers intentionality a state of mind, a mental process that can be considered synonymous with "event of consciousness." Intentionality is a basic property of the mind: it is impossible to offer a logical survey of it using simpler notions. Intentionality is a "primitive." Searle's research arises, however, in a very different perspective than that of the phenomenological tradition. Intentions are considered at the level of mind, but this consideration is carried out not through a phenomenological-transcendental investigation of consciousness, but through the analysis of human verbal behavior, linguistic and non-verbal utterances, and practical actions. Searle wants to understand intentionality's implications not only on the psychological and mental levels, as phenomenology did, but also on the linguistic and behavioral, as well as on the neurological and biological levels. The objects that for Brentano were psychic objects, and that for Husserl were acts of consciousness, the intentional *Erlebnisse*,[3] for Searle are objects of the world, of phenomenic reality: intention's directionality is directionality towards a really existing physical object, not one existing in our minds alone. We will return to this matter in the next section. For now, let us just say that almost all contemporary scholars dealing with mental processes agree that what we call consciousness is derived from physical properties of the central nervous system. Since, as we saw with Searle and Nagel, consciousness has properties that other brain functions do not possess (subjectivity, unity and intentionality), an explanation on a physical basis of consciousness is a formidable scientific problem (Kandel *et al.* 2000).

Searle and Nagel believe that consciousness is accessible to analysis through human beings' own mental processes and that so far we have been unable to realize this because it is an "emergent property" of the brain and therefore quite different from any other known cerebral property, and perhaps different from every other subject of scientific research. Among the three characteristics of consciousness, the greatest difficulties, as we have seen, are posed by subjectivity. The nature of these difficulties has been illustrated by Nagel (1995, 2012) and Searle (1998, 2010) in the following way. Suppose we manage to study the consciousness of an individual, recording the electrical activity of neurons in a given region considered important, while the subject performs a particular task requiring attention.

So far we do not know how particular cells' discharge leads to conscious perception, even in the simplest cases. According to Searle (2007), we are completely devoid of an adequate theoretical model to describe how an objective phenomenon—electrical signals in a person's brain, for instance—can create a subjective experience, as pleasure. Since consciousness is irreducibly subjective, it is beyond the scope of science as we commonly think of it. In this sense, because science is essentially a reductionist approach to the study of the events, it cannot, according to Nagel's conception (2012), address the problem of consciousness without significantly changing its methods, adopting one that allows it to demonstrate and analyze the elements of subjective experience (Kandel *et al.* 2000).

These elements are probably the basic components of cerebral functions. According to Nagel (1995, 2012), the reduction of objects to other objects does not pose any particular problems because we are able to understand, at least in principle, how the properties of a particular substance derive from the molecules that compose it.

In Nagel's point of view (1995), only after developing a theory supporting a new and fundamental type of reduction, going from the physical to the subjective, will we be able to deal with the problem of how to relate particular forms of nervous activity to particular forms of subjective experience. In order to formulate such a theory, we must first discover the building blocks of subjective consciousness. This discovery, the American philosopher says, will have an enormous impact and implications, and may require a revolution in biological thought (Nagel, 1978, 1995). However, scholars of neuroscience have been able to make significant progress in acquiring new knowledge about the neurobiology of perception without having to take into account individual experience. The avowed aim of the majority of neuroscience scholars, in fact, interested in consciousness, is more different than that outlined by philosophers of mind: their optimism regarding the eventual success of their respective undertakings derives at least partly from an interest in aspects other than those inherent in the subjective and unitary nature of consciousness (Kandel *et al.*, 2000).

It is an approach that excludes the possibility of an analysis in first person (subjective experience) in function of an explanation in reductionist terms (in third person) of the complex behaviors of the subjects studied (Weinber, 1995). In continuity with this methodology Churchland (2002, 2013; Churchland, Sejnowski, 1992) believes that if it is possible to establish a precise relationship between a particular neural event and a mental event, the description of this correlation should constitute a sufficient preliminary approximation for understanding, with a reasonable level of scientific credibility, how neural events can generate mental events. In support of this thesis, Kandel, in *Principles of Neural Science* (2000), writes:

> Having done that, we may be in a position eventually to [. . .] develop a theory of the correlations we discover empirically in order to state the *laws of correlation* between neural phenomena and subjective experience. The unitary nature of consciousness emphasized by Searle and Nagel may also not be an obstacle to fashioning a neurobiology of the mind. The unity of consciousness must depend on the brain's ability to link discrete spatial or temporal events into a single experience. [. . .] If the neural representation of a sequence like a birdsong can be successfully analyzed, why should a sequence like a sentence be, in principle, less tractable to neurobiological analysis? (Kandel *et al.*, 2000, p. 401).

Although Searle and Nagel agree with Kandel, Squire and Churchland that mental states are caused by the brain and that therefore the dualism is contradictory[4], there are still many unanswered questions:

> How exactly do neurobiological processes in the brain cause consciousness? The enormous variety of stimuli that affect us—for example, when we taste wine, look at sky, smell a rose, listen to a concert—trigger sequences of neurobiological processes that eventually cause unified, well-ordered, coherent, inner, subjective states of awareness or sentience. Now what exactly happens between the assault of the stimuli on our receptors and the experience of consciousness, and how exactly do the intermediate processes cause the conscious states?" (Searle, 1997, p. 3).

We now know, thanks to research by Kandel and Squire on the biology of memory, that what happens at the level of neurons and synapses (brain plasticity) is fundamental to the genesis of mental states, but our understanding of how this happens is very limited. We know a lot about how the brain functions, "[. . .] but we do not yet have a unifying theoretical account of how what goes on at the level of the neurobiology enables the brain to do what it does by way of causing, structuring, and organizing our mental life" (p. 198).

There are various difficulties to the development of such a theory. First and foremost there are practical problems: The brain is made up of more than 100 billion neurons connected to each other by an even higher number of connections, all in a rather narrow space, and it is difficult to work on these elements without damaging them. Nevertheless, there is no lack of neurobiologists trying to understand how mental states are caused by the brain. We can distinguish, therefore, two approaches to the problem: the particularistic or "building-block approach," and the globalistic, or "unified-field approach." The first approach considers "the entire conscious field as made up of more-or-less independent conscious units that I call 'building blocks' (Searle, 2004, p. 151); examples of these blocks are the experience of a color, a sound, a flavor. The idea behind this approach is that if we can understand how even just one of these blocks works, we would have a solution to solve the problem of mental causation as a whole. These blocks are sometimes called units or modules: "A module is a neural circuit, of differing sizes and structures in different brain regions [. . .] whose function is to receive, process and transmit neural messages" (Loeb, Poggio, 1998). The modular approach comes from observing that lesions in certain brain areas leave functions located in other areas intact. The globalistic approach, however, does not seek to understand "How does the brain produce this specific building block in the conscious field? but how does it produce the whole conscious field in the first place?" (Searle, 2004, p. 154).

Scholars do not believe that individual perceptual experiences create blocks of consciousness, but that they intervene to modify a pre-existing field of consciousness. As we saw in the second chapter, Kandel tries to combine both approaches by outlining the beginnings of an original synthesis, focused on the development of a new science of the mind that includes molecular biology (methodological reductionism) and cognitive neuroscience (holism).[5]

The study of memory is perhaps the first cognitive process to become accessible to molecular analysis. The union of molecular biology and cognitive neuroscience particularly clarifies two aspects of memory that we have considered in this work: the mnestic systems of the brain and memory storage mechanisms. Let us consider three key findings of our current scientific understanding that have emerged from the studies of mnestic systems of the brain carried out by Kandel and Squire. First, memory is composed of two basic types: declarative and non-declarative. Second, each of these two types of memory follows its own logic—conscious recollection versus unconscious memory performance. Third, each has its own neuronal system. The molecular study of the mechanisms of memory storage, in turn, has revealed surprising similarities between declarative and non-declarative memory. Both types of memory have a short-term form, lasting a few minutes, and a long-term form, lasting a few days or more. Both forms of memory, short and long-term, are based on changes in synaptic strength. Moreover, short-term storage results in only a transient change in synaptic strength. Finally, in the activation of genes and proteins is necessary to convert the short-term memory into long-term memory, in fact, storage share a common route for transmitting the signal to activate common groups of genes and proteins. Finally, both types of memory seem to grow new synapses—both of presynaptic terminals and dendritic spines—in order to stabilize long-term memory.

A further result of this synthesis is the discovery that, regardless of the brain system recruited in a particular episode of learning, the memories derived therefrom are stored in the form of changes in the strength of numerous synapses within extended groups of reciprocally connected neurons. Despite the existence of numerous types of memory, it seems that the synapses have recourse to a limited number of mechanisms, variously combined, to make these changes. Therefore, in agreement with Kandel, a memory is not determined by the type of molecules produced at the level of the synapses, but rather by the place and the nerve pathway in which the synaptic changes are made. The information stored is therefore determined by the place where the synaptic changes occur. On the contrary, the permanence of such information depends on structural changes that alter the geometry of the contacts between cells. In other words, the brain's architecture changes to be able to remember the effects of lived experiences.

Although these surprising results obtained by Kandel have allowed science to take a more elaborate and profound step forward than that made possible by genomics, conferring, perhaps permanently, an exclusive role to methodological reductionism with regard to the methods used at the level of experimental research, when instead the object of inquiry becomes the nature of consciousness and thus the framework of reference becomes a philosophical-metaphysical one, the positions of the Austrian scientist, of naturalistic and anti-dualistic inspiration, clearly show a legacy inherited from a computational outlook, closely linked to a refined form of ontological reductionism. What I mean to question here is not the idea that consciousness is a natural process that emerges from the brain, a view shared moreover by Searle and Nagel, but rather the vision[6] according to which the brain is a computational organ for processing information, whose complexity would result solely from an enormous amount of biochemical interactions, that is, from too simplistic a conception of information given the sophistication of the vital phenomena of life. This approach is derived almost exclusively from a physico-mathematical and computational context, where the concept of complexity primarily evokes computational limits, unpredictability, and sometimes, perhaps even "complications," proving furthermore to be intrinsically connected with a type of information understood as a message propagated on a carrier, after the manner of theories of computer signals or the management of digital information in general. Such a conception of organized complexity, characteristic of vital and cognitive phenomena, on the one hand irreducible to mechanistic materialism and on the other not attributable to a spiritual force, and no doubt inspired by a "physicalist" vision, is now to being revisited in light of new concepts—incompleteness, incomputability, emergence, non-linearity and semantic information—able to put ontological reductionism and biological determinism in check from within science itself. Moreover, this reconsideration of the concept is thus introducing into the context of the mind/body problem the fundamental notion of *meaningful complexity* intrinsically linked with information that is not only extensional or syntactic, but intentional in nature (Carsetti, 2009a, 2009b; Atlan, 1998). It is, thus, one of the central ideas for an embodied mind, embedded into an organism that is constantly evolving in the network of the world's and the organism's own natural processes. As we shall see shortly, cognitive activity shows itself to be "a circular process in which the defining of a single plane of knowledge inevitably creates a plurality of layers that call into question the completeness of every representation of the world. The logic of living systems transforms this incompleteness into the vital resource of the emerging plurality of cognitive strategies" (Licata, 2008).

3.2 The two faces of computationalism: symbolic and sub-symbolic systems.

If, as claimed by ontological reductionism or materialistic monism, the mind is only a set of material particles, then one can apply to it to the famous hypothesis of Laplace's Demon (1776), according to which the current state of the system of nature clearly follows from that of the previous instant. Thus if you imagine an intellect that at a given instant knew all the relationships between the entities of this universe, it could know the position, momentum and general dispositions of all these entities at any time in the past and future. Laplace proposes an interesting thought experiment. Imagine, he says, that there is a way to measure the position and velocity of all the particles of the universe. One can enter these measurements into the Newtonian mathematical framework for equations and draw out of it the fabric of the design for the entire universe, past, present and future—mind included. Naturally, Laplace knew that this hypothesis is quite similar to a computational crash; when the number of particles is very high, as for example in the theory of gases, one must resort to probability and statistics. Every irreducibility of mind to matter, every unpredictability is therefore only the expression of a practical difficulty and does not require—for the French scientist and his contemporary heirs—any additional hypothesis. From the seventeenth century to the mid-nineteenth century, the debate on the mind/body relation saw a continual oscillation between acceptance and rejection of materialism, with a number of intermediate positions.

A Copernican revolution, the true forerunner of modern cognitive science, was Kant's idea to assign mental categories the role of "organizational structures" of our perceptions, thus working a synthesis between empiricism and rationalism and giving the mind a central role in describing the world. Though space and time are the way we perceive the external world through the "channels" of mental categories, it is also true that in order to avoid idealism, which would jeopardize the possibility of a scientific description of the mind, it is necessary to admit the existence of an external world—of which the mind offers a phenomenal representation, because it is located within it. Between the eighteenth and nineteenth centuries, this rooting begins to be investigated experimentally and, thanks to the brilliant contributions of von Haller and Gall, complex interrelationships begin to be hypothesized between cognition and brain areas[7]. However, from an evolutionary point of view, one critique that can be leveled against the Kantian system is that it does not explain how the categories were formed (Licata, 2008). And so we come to what may be regarded as the inescapable question in the current debate on the essence of mind: how are mind and matter related?

To describe the processes of self-organization and emergent phenomena (such as life and mind), today the strategy that seems most effective is to refer to information. The concept of information, since its mathematical formulation in the work of Shannon as the study of the sequence of symbols transmitted over a channel between a transmitter E and a receiver R, has been of the most fruitful in modern science. Von Neumann and Wiener argued that information should be placed ideally alongside energy in the construction of scientific thought, as a quantity that can describe a system with a high degree of generality and abstraction, moreover providing an interdisciplinary language between different areas in a process of integration and unification of the sciences (von Neumann, 1958; Wiener, 1948). In the formal definition proposed by Shannon, the interest is centered on the syntactic aspects of information, with no reference to the meaning of the sequences exchanged between E and R (Shannon, 1948). This situation, although simplified, allows one to make an important connection with a key concept in the study of physical systems: Boltzmann's theory of entropy (Jaynes, 1965). This immense thermodynamic reality measures the "disorder" of a physical system through the weakening of its internal energy correlations. The increase of entropy measures the transition from a state in which the molecules are energetically bound to a precise spatial structure, to another in which they are free. In the final (asymptotic) state, there is more homogeneity and less structure. The transition to a greater level of entropy can be described as an increase in the number of microscopic configurations and a consequent loss of macroscopic structure due to lower energy correlation (increase of disorder). One of the fundamental problems of science, irresolvable within in the Newtonian mechanistic paradigm, is to understand how the tendency to disorder is compensated by the birth and development of new levels of organization. One strategy used to describe processes of self-organization is to refer to information. There is an inverse relationship between information and entropy, which builds a bridge between the notion of the organization of a system and its degree of information (Haken, 2006). As we saw in the previous paragraph, to fully understand the functioning of the biological substrates of cognitive processes, Kandel recognizes the need to go beyond the study of individual neurons and analyze the ways in which neural networks process information (Kandel, 2006). However, the computational approach he uses is not sufficient to describe the dynamics of emergent phenomena like life and the mind. The complexity of biological and cognitive processes, in fact, requires an even more sophisticated measure of information, capable of evolving by using multiple codes and modifying their semantic domains (Minati *et al.*, 2008). An exclusively syntactic theory of information is therefore insufficient to describe cognitive processes (Carsetti, 2000b). However, it is precisely in this notion that the disciplines at the origin of the science of the mind find their point of contact. The paradigm that serves as a catalyst for the meeting of the different areas is identified by Licata in the following expression: "A cognitive system is a system that processes syntactic information, a hypothesis that we shall denote by *computationalism,* a term that refers not only to information as described by Shannon, but also to a series of constraints on the informational process specified by the notions of *Turing machine* and *algorithmic procedure*" (Licata, 2008, p. 17). The connection between psychology and linguistics is a convergence between the approaches and methods of cognitivism and those of computational linguistics, where cognitive and linguistic acts are described as rules for the manipulation and production of symbols (informational blocks) whose meaning is bound by the formal structure of the symbols themselves and of the rules adopted. This finds correspondence in the information sciences, whose role is not only to investigate the mathematical procedures for processing information, but also to provide experimental devices to test the hypothesis of the computational mind: computers. Though the mind can be described as a syntactic information processor, it is still largely independent of the material structure that supports it. An abstract and disembodied vision of the mind, therefore, is at the origin of the adventure of *artificial intelligence.* The computationalism that inspired the birth of cognitive science, then, can be considered the direct expression of the Platonic soul in science and of Hilbert's formalist programmer in the foundations of mathematics. "The paradoxical aspect of the story is that precisely Gödel's and Turing's limiting results of the formalist programmer would produce the computer and that particular type of computationalism that uses the idea of the *computer as a metaphor for the mind*" (pp. 19–20).

The limitations of the symbolic approach, identified by the failures of artificial intelligence, have ensured that especially since the eighties we have developed a different strategy to attack the problem of cognition; we are referring to the sub-symbolic or connectionist approach, whose typical examples are the numerous classes of neural networks (Grossberg, 1988; Hopfield, 1982). Here, the Aristotelian soul and the procedural aspect prevail, since the essential idea is that mental activity described "macroscopically" through symbolic systems (mathematics, language, etc.) actually emerges from the cooperative behavior of many constituent units whose microscopic patterns may vary in relation to precisely those dynamic processes that had proved taboo for symbolic computationalism, namely learning, image recognition and more generally the procedures which in some way involve a modification of the semantic domain of the system (Pessa, Penna, 1994). The methodology used by sub-symbolic systems is that of dynamic systems, or systems of differential equations that describe the spatio-temporal evolution of a network structure composed of nodes (formal neurons) and connections between nodes (synapses). Each node is characterized by a degree of activation, i.e., a threshold value beyond which the neuron becomes sensitive to external stimuli and lights up. Finally, each connection is associated with a numerical coefficient (weight) that regulates the transmission of the activation. The deformation of the network in its various dynamic configurations (patterns) can be considered as the geometric expression of its learning. In this way, symbolic knowledge is fragmented in distributed and parallel configurations that emerge from the collective behavior of elements of micro-cognition (Licata, 2011).

The advantage of the sub-symbolic systems over those of the symbolic type consists, as is evident, of their greater flexibility and complexity in processing information: the activity of a network is parallel and not sequential, the problem of an input-output error in a single unit therefore does not decisively affect the final result. Another advantage consists in the fact that the network models are immersed in a much more varied external environment of stimuli than the purely formal environment of symbolic systems. It is wrong however to say that the networks are more realistic from the biological point of view. This is because the type of information involved is essentially the same as that of symbolic systems and the system is passive with respect to the flow of information and the external environment, just as in symbolic systems. And here lies, in my opinion, the fundamental limitation of Kandel's approach. The current models of networks are not able to produce high forms of hierarchical organization, that is, they are not capable of "abstraction" in analyzing configurations. It therefore seems that the symbolic systems and those based on micro-cognition possess complementary properties: the former are easier to organize hierarchically but extremely rigid, the latter show a great deal of flexibility but have a limit of structural complexity. Also, at a deeper level there is the problem of the unidimensionality of information in both types of systems. Both cases involve syntactic information managed according to a Turing-style computational model of an algorithmic kind (Turing, 1950). "This means that the limit of both systems consists ultimately in a description of system-environment relations through a fixed pattern, which does not generate new codes and therefore is structurally incapable of abstraction and intentionality, and of displaying genuine autonomy. These issues reveal the gap between artificial systems and natural knowledge" (Licata, 2008, p. 20).

The proposed approaches, therefore, have as a sub-goal and constraint the hypothesis that an intelligent system can be designed and in some cases actually built. This follows directly from computationalism's theoretical apparatus and from the close interaction between theory and technology in the development of artificial intelligence systems and devices based on neural architecture. There are two currents within traditional artificial intelligence, commonly called *strong artificial intelligence* and *weak artificial intelligence* (Pessa, 1992). The first argues that a symbolic processing system can think; indeed, it has to. What it should think about depends simply on the complexity of the system and the programs that make it work. *A priori,* there is no reason not to believe that one day we will be able to build a program that allows a computer to think like a human being, but our comparison of man and computer is based solely on outwardly observable behavior and it concerns rules for the manipulation of symbols. Weak artificial intelligence, instead, recognizes that the issue of thought transcends the current ideas inspired by the proper logic of the computer sciences. At the same time, however, it considers symbolic processing programs useful in providing models of cognitive processes (Pessa, 1993; Penna, Pessa, 1998).

Strong artificial intelligence was refuted in 1980 by Searle, with his famous "Chinese Room" argument (Searle, 1984). Given that the written Chinese language is not alphabetic, but ideographic, that is, every word, or every concept, is represented by a single ideogram, Searle imagines an individual placed in a room, who does not know Chinese and has boxes full of Chinese characters and a manual written in a language known by the individual, which explains how to relate the input characters with other characters for output. Outside the room are people who know Chinese; they insert characters into the room and interpret the output characters produced by the individual, who from within the room manipulates them according to the rules in the manual. Since the manual is written in such a way that the output ideograms are indistinguishable from responses furnished by a native Chinese person, people outside the room will have no way of knowing that the individual inside does not know Chinese, since the responses obtained from their questions are identical to those a Chinese person would provide. Yet the individual does not know Chinese at all and is, by definition, utterly incapable of understanding the meaning of the ideograms he manipulates. Therefore, understanding Chinese, as well as any other cognitive activity, cannot in any way be reduced to the manipulation of symbols according to the rules of a "symbolic" processing program (Searle, 1984; Penna, Pessa, 1998).

What Searle's argument means to highlight is the difference between syntax (grammar) and semantics. Thought is essentially based on semantics, which can never be expressed in purely symbolic terms, because it requires connections between the world of symbols and that of real facts, a relationship which is foreign to symbolic processing. The only change necessary in order for symbols to produce concrete objects or events, is that there be a real mediator (a living being), effecting these changes. In Searle's eyes, it is impossible for a purely symbolic processing system to think, as strong artificial intelligence claims, because thought is a direct product of the relationship between a real biological brain and the meaningful environment (the world of events surrounding it) (Searle, 1998). In conclusion, Searle's reasoning undermines not only strong artificial intelligence, but also any theory of mind of the computational symbolic type, such as that of Fodor (1975, 1983), putting in crisis every computational and symbolic theory of mind. According to the American philosopher the Chinese room argument also works against the paradigm of sub-symbolic processing upheld by connectionism (Searle, 1984, 1997, 2001). He, in fact, generalized the Chinese room argument, positing a scenario in which there isn't just one person in the room, but a group of people who share ideograms according to precise processing rules, just as the units of a neural network do when exchanging signals. Also in this case, the conclusions are not far from the precedent, because it is impossible to assert either that the individual people know Chinese, or that the group of people as a whole knows it: even a neural network is incapable of thought. In other words, Searle bases his argument on the assumption that a connectionist model is computationally equivalent to a traditional model of symbolic processing (Pessa, Penna, 2004), because the majority of neural networks are simulated on traditional computers, using old programs. The result is that, at a qualitative level, the paradigm of sub-symbolic processing is substantially equivalent to that of computational symbolic processing, because it is incapable of giving rise to semantics[8] (Pessa, Penna, 1994).

In conclusion, to understand in depth the complex logic underlying the neurophysiological mechanisms involved in memory, learning, linguistic and sensory-motor activities, it is necessary to go beyond Kandel's conception that the brain is merely a computational processing system, and to identify new non-reductionist and non-deterministic models of gene expression and synaptic interaction also capable of dealing fully with the concepts of function and meaning. At this level it will be possible to consider the human brain as a complex system capable of generating ever new information.

3.3 Complex systems and biological information

One conceptual aspect of reductionism is the idea that the world is "already there," clearly organized from the smallest to the most complex levels, and that the latter are composed only by intricate expression of the interactions of a large number of elementary objects. This neat simplicity captures only a small part of the world we live in and the majority of highly complex systems cannot be explained by such an approach, while remaining invisible to a reductionist investigation (Licata, 2011).

In 1963 an event took place that would soon change significantly the way of looking at reality in all the sciences, including physics: Edward Lorenz discovered deterministic chaos, whose foundations had been laid already by Poincaré in 1889 with the three body problem. Lorenz showed that a very simple model of nonlinear differential equations was sufficient to produce chaotic behavior in a dynamic system. In this case, despite the rigorous determinism of Newton's law, one observes the presence of chaotic behavior in the system, caused by the extreme sensitivity of the solutions to the equations at the initial conditions (Barrow-Green, 1997). It happens that two states, no matter how similar to each other, come to distance themselves exponentially over time. From the impossibility, both in practice and in principle, of defining the initial conditions with infinite precision, there follows a substantial unpredictability of the state of the system, which becomes less and less controllable the greater the time that has elapsed from the initial instant.

And thus, in all disciplines of the sixties and seventies, new languages were born, capable of representing the properties of systems characterized by a functional and structural complexity that prevents one from deducing them from those of their components. These languages are based on the inadequacy of considering reductionism the only valid scientific method, and accept the irreducibility of the different levels of organization of such systems and the inability to find complete explanations of their properties without resorting to historical and evolutionary categories (biological organisms, the mind, memory, the immune system, social organization, economies). This new way of investigating reality, which some scholars call the "challenge of complexity," leads us to believe that simple phenomena, manifestations of universal natural laws, which in classical science were the rule, are actually rare exceptions (Bocchi, Ceruti, 2007). All this requires, then, a new characterization of time: time in classical and relativistic mechanics is a simple variable in the equations of motion, it flows evenly and doesn't bring about novelties, since all the information is contained in the initial conditions. Today, however, a new concept of time is emerging, since the majority of chemical, physical and biological phenomena cannot be explained in terms of "laws" but of "processes," where time is always the bearer of new information, because in time the "choices" of the system are determined, which constitute its "history," according to an evolution that is unpredictable from the initial conditions (Prigogine, 1980; Prigogine, Stengers, 1979; Nicolis, Prigogine, 1989).

Ilya Prigogine, the Nobel Prize winner in science in 1977, was responsible for applying complex systems to biology; in particular, he was involved in the study of ordered systems in non-equilibrium. One example of a continuous structure in non-equilibrium is the Great Red Spot of Jupiter, which is essentially a system of storms that have been present for several centuries. It is a stable organization of matter and energy through which both flow. Its similarity with a human organism, whose molecular components change many times during the course of its life, is impressive. Thermodynamic systems in non-equilibrium, thus, are powered by the constant dissipation of matter and energy; for this reason Prigogine named them dissipative structures, systems in which the flow of matter and energy becomes a driving force capable of generating order: this is a paradoxical state of affairs that challenges our intuitions about the behavior of large populations (Nicolis, Prigogine,

1977). The chaos that is indifferent to equilibrium is followed by a "creative chaos," similar to that evoked by some Presocratics, a fertile chaos, which can potentially yield different structures (Prigogine, Stengers, 1979). Living systems, therefore, according to Prigogine, are dissipative structures (complex metabolic vortices). Cells, in fact, are dissipative structures in non-equilibrium: complex chemical systems that continually metabolize nutritive molecules to maintain their internal structure and reproduce. Equilibrium means death for most cells. Prigogine thus sees a close link between self-organization and a system's distance from equilibrium. Life, however, constitutes an exceptional state of matter: it may well be that order, coherency, are located in a certain sense between "equilibrium thermal chaos" and "non-equilibrium turbulent chaos." However, these two types of disorder are very different. "In thermal chaos as realized in equilibrium, all characteristic space and time scales are of molecular range, while in turbulent chaos we have such an abundance of macroscopic time and length scales that the system appears chaotic" (Prigogine, Stengers, 1984, p. 168). From this perspective, life with its characteristic coherency seems to belong to a kind of intermediary system. The distance from balance is sufficient but not excessive, so as to avoid the destruction of the delicate configuration necessary to maintain the normal life functions (Prigogine, Stengers, 1988). The living state of matter is thus a transitional state between order and chaos: life emerges right on the edge of chaos, where matter becomes able to perceive and communicate (Kauffman, 1993). Life, therefore, is located in an intermediate state between the order of a crystal and the disorder of a smoke ring; it is there that complex behaviors emerge (Atlan, 1987). With Prigogine's studies a new science began, which some scholars call the science of complexity (Nicolis, Prigogine, 1989; Prigogine, 1993). It would be developed within biology in the nineties thanks to the considerable contribution made by biochemist S. Kauffman's research carried out at the Santa Fe Institute. The American scholar writes in his 1995 book *At Home in The Universe. The Search of the Laws of Self-Organization and Complexity:* "Just between [order and chaos], just near this phase transition, just at the edge of chaos, the most complex behaviors can occur—orderly enough to ensure stability, yet full of flexibility and surprise. Indeed, this is what we mean by complexity" (Kauffman, 1995, p. 46). In the context of complexity theory, therefore, in agreement with Kauffman, life—just like cognition—appears as

> an emergent phenomenon arising as the molecular diversity of a non-living chemical system increases beyond a threshold of complexity. If true, then life is not located in the property of any single molecule—in the details—but is a collective property of systems of interacting molecules. Life, in this view, emerged whole and has always remained whole. [. . .] No vital force or extra substance is present in the emergent, self-reproducing whole. But the collective system does possess a stunning property not possessed by any of its parts. It is able to reproduce itself and to evolve. The collective system is alive. Its parts are just chemicals" (p. 15).

Thus, we can say that biological or cognitive systems are systems that are complex, non-linear (unpredictable), dissipative (they exchange energy with the outside), capable of generating information (from the chaos, order is generated): in chaotic dynamics you can separate the energy fluxes from the information fluxes, they are independent of each other (Shaw, 1981). Though relevant in a logical and physical-mathematical context, the notion of "information," like that of "complexity," takes on richer implications in biology. To speak of information is to speak of immaterial form, a concept clearly present in the Aristotelian philosophy of nature, then interpreted in the Stagirite's metaphysics as one of the four causes of being: the formal cause. In contrast with what Kandel, Squire, Churchland and Damasio claim, here information is not just a message that propagates itself on a support, as in theories of computer signals or in general in information management; rather it means actualization, the ability to inform through a form, by not only dropping information into matter, but actualizing the matter itself, to make it what it should be. The universe is a universe of forms, a world where information is irreducible to matter (understood as mass + energy) but is also actualized in matter and "causes matter to be" (Tanzella-Nitti, 2009; Basti, 2011). An observation that inevitably leads to the important question about the origin of information.

Fruitful, here, are the reflections that the philosopher accustomed to the Aristotelian scheme could then make about the link between formal cause and final cause—which the Stagirite saw as being in close relationship, the form containing the information about the purpose. Cognitive systems, therefore, are complex systems that constantly generate new information. In these circumstances, the emergence of consciousness, within the context of the mind/body problem, cannot simply be explained by the use of known forms of materialistic monism[9] like behaviorism, physicalism, computationalism (or strong AI) and the more extreme "eliminative materialism" according to which phenomena or mental states do not exist at all (Searle, 1992), but can be "interpreted" as an order that, emerging from chaos, can self-assemble in ever different ways, also producing a different type of information no longer measurable by Shannon's and Wiener's traditional theory, which is based on an overly simplistic mathematical model (Shannon, 1948).

In recent years, a new physics of emergence has developed whose job it is to investigate the intertwined hierarchies of the evolution of complex systems. The notion of emergence has been developed by studying phase transitions and collective processes, providing powerful mathematical tools that have allowed researchers to shed light at last on the age-old epistemological question concerning the relationship between mind and world (Vitiello, 2004, 2009b; Vitiello, Pessa, 2003; Freeman, Vitiello, 2008, 2009). Indeed, an understanding of cognitive processes today requires a new kind of scientific explanation in which the goal is no longer to reduce these processes to key components and manage to predict events with precision, but is rather to discover the conditions under which a process can actually emerge. "The central idea is that the more complex a system is, the greater the perspectives from which it can be observed, showing aspects and organizational levels that cannot be broken down neatly and solved by a single model based on a single, fundamental equation that is so important in traditional systems of physics. Complexity requires the viewer to employ a variety of approaches in his investigation, none of which by itself provides a definitive explanation" (Licata, 2008, p. xiii).

In this way the observer and his cognitive strategies become an integral part of the theory and the sought-after unity between physics and cognition occurs in an epistemological project on the dialogic relations between the observer and the observed. Turing computing, the model of the digital computer, is abstract and disembodied, while natural computation (biological information) considers the processing of information to be a process closely related to the physical structure of the system that performs the computing. In these systems with an extremely open logic, a cognitive domain appears, i.e., the ability to produce and manage information in an autonomous way and generally one that is irreducible to a single formal model (semantic emergence). This is one of the central ideas for an embodied mind, embedded in an organism that is constantly evolving in the network of natural processes (Varela *et al.*, 1991; Varela, 1997, 1999). Cognitive activity shows itself thus to be "a circular process in which the defining of a single plane of knowledge inevitably creates a plurality of layers that call into question the completeness of every representation of the world" (Licata, 2008, p. XII). The open logic of living systems transforms this incompleteness into the vital resource for the emerging plurality of cognitive strategies. What, then, are the principles underlying the genesis of life forms and their self-organization, a self-organization that is much more complex than that manifested by an atmospheric disturbance or by other not-yet-living natural phenomena?

Some possible answers to this question might be found in the revisiting carried out, above all, by J. Hintikka (1970) on the concept of semantic information, as outlined originally by Carnap and Bar Hillel in 1952, through the development in the sixties and seventies of a theory of depth information that has significantly broadened the horizon of Carnap's original assumptions, to the point of facing the same problem of finding a possible determination of the content of semantic information at the level of polyadic structures. Almost simultaneously, in the seventies and eighties, algorithmic information theory, on the basis of the original studies of Kolmogorov and Chaitin, was outlining its theoretical connotations with particular regard to the issues of incompleteness and incompressibility, coming finally to a precise re-examination of Gödel's original findings (Kolmogorov, 1965; Chaitin, 1987, 1990).

These theoretical developments were soon to be grafted onto the issues of cognitivism and connectionism: the result was the real possibility of a new approach to delineate the path of the construction of knowledge, an approach capable of taking into account, in a significant manner, that particular interweaving of incompressibility, on the one hand, and meaning on the other, that constitutes the connective tissue of the human mind. This approach resulted in the birth of a specific version of complexity theory in the nineties, able to take into account the problem of the very constitution, throughout the course of natural and cultural evolution, of the mental operations that characterize objective knowledge (Carsetti, 1984b, 1989, 1991). Of course, the link between evolution and entropy must be seen in relation to complex biosystems becoming real, biosystems endowed with an internal code, specific apparatuses of rules and the capacity for self-programming. It is necessary, in this sense, to go beyond Shannon's characterization of the concept of information.

According to Carsetti (1987) our ability to arrive at distinguishing microstates able to account for the articulation of an entropic function linked to specific regulatory constraints of a biological character can allow us to outline an explanation, in general, of the processes of threshold and self-organization proper to cognitive systems. In other words, it is necessary first of all to realize that we cannot calculate biological information the way we do the transmission of signals. It is not sufficient to take account of the intervention of the measuring activity, distinguishing free information from information which is linked, when we are unable to locate the intrinsic reality of biological microstates and, therefore, the type of constraints specific to them. It is necessary, instead, in Carsetti's eyes, to find the levels of depth information, where the regulatory constraints are hidden; it is furthermore necessary to account for the relationship joining the observer to the source, and in particular, to explain the link between the various levels at which the content of information is located (Carsetti 1989).

As Jaynes (2000) rightly noted, going into deeper levels of the source, in this case the brain, is only possible with the help of very sophisticated telescopes/models, with the help of measures of information and hypotheses that are not rigidly predetermined. Measures and hypotheses that are able, we should add, to explain the complex interplay between surface information and depth information, to account for how noise, generated primarily at the internal level, can be used in a creative way and become a driver of innovation. What we have said so far can be broadly summarized, according to Carsetti, by saying that a process of self-organization suitable to determine the "qualitative" growth of the system's own complexity, may actually occur only where the active presence of certain background factors is ensured: a) the coupled character of the global system: the presence, that is to say, of a continuous interaction between source and observer; b) the interwoven articulation of a multiplicity of processes of reflection, invention and selection; c) the presence of an autonomous code inside the source (system of instructions), designed to ensure that while the source expresses itself, at the same time, it specifies its own structure; d) an independent development of the system that is woven according to the characteristics of a real evolutive tinkering; e) the presence, on the one hand, of latent potential at the source level of releasing possible factors, and the presence at the level of the observer, on the other hand, of specific programs of factors, namely, intervention, reflection and coagulum (Carsetti, 1987, 1989). Within this framework, therefore, in our view, it is important to possess a theory of information that not focuses only on the determination of particular distributions of probability, on the one hand, and on the determination of the conditions of ergodicity, on the other, but that also defines the content of "structure-object" type information determined in terms of the complexity of the objects themselves, of the amount of information necessary to calculate and generate the structures in question. Well, the concept provided by Shannon does not allow one to analyze sample points beyond the surface level, as these are defined, moreover, in relation to a network of constraints of a Markovian character that limits, in turn, these points' relational possibilities, as well as the range of choice related thereto (Carsetti, 1987).

Today there is an urgent need for a theory of self-organization capable, ultimately, of being articulated at an intentional and hyper-intentional level. It is necessary, in fact, to extend the standard framework in regard to traditional Boolean models, to build a new and more general type of theoretical concept: the concept of a self-organizing model. The theoretical core of this new concept is represented by the intuition that the terrain of semantics is not constituted by domains of atomic individuals, but by information flows, that is, by generative and recurring processes (Carsetti, 1999). These processes determine a clear hierarchy of levels characterized in an intentional way. The processes of self-organization, in agreement with Carsetti (2000b), should be considered, firstly, as a sort of teleonomic "arch," able to join meaningful complexity and selection by elimination. In this context, the selection by the meaning can show itself to be autonomous primarily to the extent that it proves capable of "modulating" the continuous irruption of new generative apparatuses (Carsetti, 2009a). To elaborate a theory of biological information (or natural computation) that is able to deal with the intentional complexity of the human mind, therefore, we need to build a new process semantics applicable to biology, i.e., a semantics that is no longer just of the interpretative kind, but rather of the generative kind. There has been a request from scientists in various fields to define the principles of a new algorithmic information theory, not exclusively anchored to a propositional base, but articulated at the level or dimension of a predicative and stratified logic. Compared to such a theoretical framework, in agreement with Carsetti, the real problem is to "follow" the real contours of the generative and productive dynamic's evolution at work in order to trigger, on the real level, a real deployment of depth information and not to identify each time the different possible compromises between fluctuations, on the one hand, and stabilization processes, on the other. In this sense, then, the construction of new algorithms able to describe the invention of further cognitive models will present itself as one of the essential steps for achieving a better understanding of the complexity of living systems and, at the same time, a richer articulation of their potential to evolve (Carsetti, 2010a).

Since the end of the last century, the current research into cognitive function, as we have seen, has in the broadest sense been moving away from the computational matrix which had originally generated such research, drawing ever closer to an interpretation of the mind (and its cognition) as "embodied," situated and distributed. A mind that no longer resides only in the individual, but also in individuals, in the contexts that live and transform themselves; a mind that can no longer be studied separately, in itself, but in an increasingly integrated way, by considering the dynamic unity of its parts correlating it to the brain, to the body, and making it, together with them, an organism, in the same way we ought to consider "organismic" its synergistic and interactive situation with the environment, which includes it, contains it and, at the same time, specifies and distinguishes it. Consequently, the idea that a cognitive agent is something centralized and unified (phrenology's notion of "localization") has been replaced by the concept of a "dis-unified" self. The modules, in fact, are incomprehensible to cognitive experience and lack access to consciousness and introspection. From here it emerges that the cognitive self is not represented by a totality, but by a series of emerging units from this "dis-unified" network (Zeki, 1999). The cognitive process, thus, now reveals itself as an emergence of form and not the shaping of form. It is unpredictable morphogenesis, and not a program, reducible to algorithmic procedures (Sabatano, 2004; Frauenfelder *et al.*, 2004). Scientific research must, therefore, head in the direction of a globality in which the cognitive does not prevail over the relational but where, on the contrary, the relational channel becomes a participant in strategic operations and in operations of organizing and selecting through the information mass (Bruner, 1993). Today like never before the problem of knowledge is a problem of the person with his history, his conscience, and never has the problem of knowledge been so highly complex (Sabatano, 2004).

The fundamental contribution of a theory of biological information to epistemology lies in describing in wholly general terms the relationship between observer and observed as an adaptive and co-evolutionary intentional process, where the ability to construct models of the world appears as a search for connections with an ever-wider degree of openness. In this sense, complexity theory is a "theory of everything" in a much more ambitious sense than that of physicists, as it allows you to frame in a single logical schema the relationship between mind and world, and constitutes the formal core of a new *Physis* able to understand mind and matter as dynamic elements of a unitary scenario (Atlan, 2000; Davies, Gregersen, 2010).

In these last few years, therefore, cognitive science, neurobiology, quantum mechanics, biomathematics and bioinformatics, on the one hand, and functional semantics, non-standard semantics and symbolic dynamics, on the other, have led to the progressive opening of new and fruitful horizons of research also with regard to the scope of complexity theory, that is, the interdisciplinary study of complex adaptive systems (natural and biological systems) and the emergent phenomena associated with them, whose articulation has continued to expand—thanks to the considerable contribution of scholars such as Freeman, Atlan and Carsetti—no longer referring to the simple analysis of dissipative phenomena of a Markovian mold, and going so far as to examine the phenomena of the elaboration and coupled transformation of information, phenomena which are present at the level of the subsequent formation of a biological system for processing information itself. Thus Kandel's and Squire's methodological reductionism has come to be flanked by a holistic view not rooted in the vital spirit, but in mathematics itself, in which biological systems are neither equivalent to the sum of their parts, nor determinable solely on the basis of the initial conditions. Cognitive systems, in fact, as affirmed by Atlan (1987, 2000) and Carsetti (1991, 1999, 2000a), are characterized by the fact that what self-organizes within them is the very function that determines them and their meaning. We can recognize here that particular mix of complexity, self-organization, emergence and intentionality that characterizes the natural forms of the cognitive activity of every living system. In this context, therefore, the study of the mechanisms of the transmission of information, at the basis of the mind's processes of self-organization, is undertaken through new mathematical models no longer linked to the instruments offered by Shannon's traditional information theory, or by Boolean algebra, or Halmos's, or by Markov's processes. A cognitive science that wants to go beyond reductionism, therefore, will have to confront depth information, meaning that creative and organizing function that responds to a mathematics in many ways still undiscovered, able to give an account of those highly complex, unpredictable phenomena, not yet the subject of a known method of measurement.[10] According to Atlan (1985, 1987), models of self-organization allow us to see in living organisms no longer a kind of deterministic automata directed by a program supplied from the outside, in the manner of today's computers (think BCI techniques), but self-organizing systems whose principles are beginning to spread among researchers in the field of artificial intelligence.

> The most important of the phenomena of self-organization is the creation of new meanings in the information transmitted from one part to another of the organism, or from one level of organization to another level of organization. For disorganization to be able to produce a reorganization, it is necessary for the meaning of the relationships between the parts to be transformed. This is why the question of the creation of meanings is located at the center of the phenomena of self-organization (Atlan, 1985, p. 143).

3.4 The pre-conditions of ethics

In the introduction of his 1797 masterpiece the *Metaphysics of Morals*, Immanuel Kant offers a definition of life: "The capacity of a being to act in accordance with its representations is called *life*" (Kant, 1797, p. 211). At first glance it seems that this phrase refers only to persons endowed with consciousness, when in reality, if you revisit this wonderful definition in the light of contemporary life sciences, some original aspects are sure to emerge. For example, more than two hundred years since Kant's brilliant words, systemic biology cannot but acknowledge in the great philosopher of the eighteenth century the merit of having identified one of the main features of *bios:* cognition. But that is not all: soon it becomes clear how, in living organisms, cognition is deeply linked to the fundamental notion of intentionality.

In his book, *Darwin's Dangerous Idea,* Dennett proposes a hierarchy of forms of knowledge arising during evolution by Darwinian means. He distinguishes between *Darwinian creatures, Pavlovian creatures, Popperian creatures* and *Gregorian creatures.* "A variety of candidate organisms were blindly generated by more or less arbitrary processes of recombination and mutation of genes. These organisms were field-tested, and only the best designed survived. This is the ground floor of the Tower. Let us call its inhabitants *Darwinian creatures*" (Dennett, 1995, p. 374). An autonomous agent as simple as, for example, a bacterium is a Darwinian creature. In its simplest version, such a creature evolves by mutation, but also by recombination and natural selection (without considering any behavioral learning). Therefore, a creature, a colony or an ecosystem will adapt itself roughly as Darwin thought. "These individuals thus confronted the environment by generating a variety of actions, which they tried out, one by one, until they find one that worked. We may call this subset of Darwinian creatures, the creatures with conditionable plasticity, Skinnerian creatures" (p. 374). Then, in the level above that of Darwinian creatures, according to Dennet, there is a nervous system, and the creature (for example, the Aplysia) is capable of stimulus-response learning. In actual fact, the Aplysia can learn simple conditioned stimuli; the most recent analogy is the bell that causes the dog to salivate in expectation of food. "Skinnerian conditioning is a fine capacity to have, so long as you are not killed by one of your early errors. A better system involves pre-selection among all the possible behaviors or actions, weeding out the truly stupid ones before risking them in the harsh world [. . .].

We may call the beneficiaries of this third story in the Tower Popperian creatures, since, as Sir Karl Popper once elegantly put it, this design enhancement 'permits our hypotheses to die in our stead'" (p. 375). According to Dennett, then, Popperian creatures—we vertebrates—have internal models of our world and can freely manipulate the internal model, rather than activating the model in real time in the real world. In this way, then, just as Popper said, "our hypotheses die in our stead." "The successors of simple Popperian creatures are those whose inner environments are permeated by parts designed by the external environment. The creatures of this sub-sub-subset might be called Gregorian creatures, as the British psychologist Richard Gregory is in my opinion the preeminent theorist of the role of information [. . .] in the creation of shrewd moves" (p. 377). We humans are Gregorian creatures. Dennett's reasoning is very simple: we use our tools (stone knives, arrows, farming tools, machine tools) to expand our world of facts and processes. This shared, widened world provides us with more know-how and more knowledge. At some point, however, cultural evolution breaks loose: rock music, for example, invades Iranian minarets. In continuity with what has been said so far, moreover, as the great scientist Kauffman commented:

> I very much like Dennett's ladder of know-how, and eventual know that. Without invoking consciousness, not because it is

> not worth invoking but because so little that is sensible has been said on the subject, it seems worth asking how much of this hierarchy could be realized by simple molecular systems, even without evoking nerve cells. [. . .] For example, bacteria and amoebae do have a kind of Pavlovian learning already, [. . .] This is not yet the association of a more or less arbitrary conditioned stimulus with an unconditioned stimulus, but I can imagine chemistry to accomplish the latter. As neurons are supposed to proliferate and form novel synaptic connections that survive if used and to mediate the linkage of conditioned to unconditioned stimulus, why not envision a complex chemistry, say, very complex carbohydrate-synthesis patterns sustained by complex sets of enzymes whose activities are modulated by the different carbohydrates themselves [. . .] The image is not too far from how it is imagined that 'idiotype' and 'anti-idiotype' immune networks work to sustain synthesis of a set of desired antibodies against an incoming pathogen. In such networks, for which there is modestly good evidence, a given first antibody serves as an antigen that stimulates the body to produce a second antibody that binds to the unique amino acid sequences ('idiotype') of the first antibody [. . .] In conclusion the biologist observes that it is reasonable to think of the immune system as a conditioned stimulus response system" (Kauffman, 2005, pp. 115–116).

Consider, for example, Dennett's Popperian creatures: do they have to have nerves? It appears that plants send each other signals using complex secondary metabolites, to characterize the kinds of insects that infest the clearing. Between the metabolite and the insect, arbitrary structural relationships are established, just as the symbols of human language are often arbitrary with respect to the thing signified. Not bad for invertebrates with no nervous system. But let us move on, now, to consider Gregorian creatures.

> Even here, the free and open creating of new symbol strings in a language, wherever new sentences can be created, is not that fundamentally different from the persistent open creation of new

> kinds of molecules in the biosphere as a whole. [. . .] I suppose I am naively driven to consider that the biosphere, with its urgent diversity in which, emboldened by all our know-how, we do get on with a very rich conversation, may very early already have harbored all the levels of which Dennet speaks (p. 116).

Posed in these terms, know-how, according to Kauffman, is another way of viewing the catalytic closures that propagate themselves, the work tasks, perception, the recording and the actions, which we now recognize as inherent in the activities of autonomous agents.[11] The know-how is not outside the processes of self-organization: know-how is organization propagating itself. In this respect, therefore, in the eyes of the great American scholar, with autonomous agents also comes a glimmer of an ethical issue.

> The emergence of ethics in the evolution of life on this planet is a fascinating issue. I will content myself with wondering where 'value' and the rudiments of 'intentionality' come from in the physical universe [. . .]. Facts are know-that statements. But know-how preceded know that. While fully aware of Hume's injunction, I think that from the autonomous agent's perspective, yuck or yum is primary, unavoidable, and of the deepest importance to that agent. I suppose we apply the Darwinian criteria. Too much yuck, this one and its progeny are gone from the future of the biosphere. Without attributing consciousness to an *E. coli,* or an autonomous agent we may create in the near future, I cannot help but feel that the rudiments of value are present once autonomous agents are around" (pp. 116–117).

Let us return for a moment to Kant's definition. Life understood as the power to act in a manner consistent with one's own representations not only tells us that all living beings are cognitive systems, but also tells us that these bodies act according to internal models, creating in this way ever new meanings. From a phenomenological point of view, a representation can be read as a re-presentation of something. The term "representation," therefore, implicitly contains the inside/

outside distinction and thus directionality towards external reality perceived through interior status changes that can be answered through simple actions. We believe that this tension towards exteriority, which Kant alone intuited, can be defined as intentionality without any reference to consciousness, that is, as the process, closely connected to the gratuitousness of molecular interactions, by which meanings are developed and, once embodied in action, operate, also allowing autonomous agents to change for their own benefit the environment in which they live, in order to reproduce. Think for a moment of the humble *E. coli* that swims upstream in a glucose gradient. The bacterium is an autocatalytic system[12] able to reproduce and thus act by performing one or more cycles of thermodynamic work, but it is also a cognitive system capable of creating ever new meanings and, subsequently, of transmitting them by means of non-conscious actions. Bacteria and amoebae, as we know, already manifest a learning that we could describe as Pavlovian, to use Dennett's terminology; these organisms have receptors that adapt on a constant level of a certain ligand-signal and that perceive a change from the present level: behold, thus, the emergence in biology of a primitive form (unconscious, of course) of representation. Here, therefore, though we cannot yet speak of association between a more or less arbitrary conditioned stimulus and an unconditioned stimulus, it is still possible to infer that these organisms are to all effects endowed with that four-billion-year-old faculty which Kauffman defines as know-how, intentionality without reference to consciousness. At this point, therefore, the brilliance of Kant's intuition becomes evident: "The capacity of a being to act in accordance with its representations is called *life*." Something remains to be clarified, however, in this definition. What is meant by the term "act"? In the attempt to give an initial response to this question, it seems useful to examine attentively Kauffman's thought: he makes a distinction between the 'doings' of an autonomous agent (agency) and mere happenings in and around the autonomous agent. In the American biologist's opinion this kind of difference is relevant for autonomous agents in general. In this sense, he argues that the rudiments of semantics as well as intentionality, value and ethics arise with autonomous agents (Kauffman, 2005).

Thus, the fundamental difference between what is alive and what is not resides in the ability to act, that is, in that process that allows meaning to manifest itself in time. That process derives from agency. In another brilliant insight, Kauffman informs us that the simple swimming or orienting of a bacterium toward an increased rate of glucose molecules (detected by the bacterium's glucose receptor) is an interpreted sign that allows the bacterium to move up the glucose gradient (Kauffman, 2008).

> Without agency, as far as I can tell, there can be no meaning. It is a very long distance to human agency and meaning. But it is we humans who *use* the computer to solve *our* problems. It is we who invest meanings in the physical states of the water bowls or electronic states of the silicon chip. This meaning is the semantics missing in the Turing machine's computations. Without the semantics the Turing machine is merely a set of physical states of marks on paper [. . .] Similarly, it is not a wonder than Shannon brilliantly *ignored semantics* to arrive at his quantitative theory of the amount of information carried down a channel. That is why Shannon tells us the *amount of information* passing down a channel, a syntactic quantity, but does not tell us what information *is*" (Kauffman, 2008, p. 193).

Kauffman's words make it clear that autonomous agents constitute that mysterious place of physics where physics is open to semantics; but in my opinion, we must distinguish on the scale of living beings the actions of simple autonomous agents, such as amoebas and bacteria, and of more complex ones, such as tigers and chimpanzees, from those of *Homo sapiens,* to date the only known species capable of good and evil. With *Homo sapiens,* there makes its appearance on earth the most deeply teleonomic nervous system that has ever existed in the history of our biosphere: only at this level, then, is nature, becoming aware of itself, actually able to transform meaningful actions into freely willed acts.

To understand fully the scope of these considerations, it seems necessary to invoke Kant's aid once more, who in the *Metaphysics of Morals* distinguishes with great insight the term "action" (*Handlung*) from that of "act" (*That*). An action (*Handlung*) constitutes a change set in motion by the subject, or by any living being; an act (*that*), however, is the material content of the action, that is, that of which the subject is the author (Kant, 1797, p. 223). According to Kant, then, only man performs acts because man alone, as the only self-conscious being, is able to recognize an action responsibly as an expression of his own subjectivity. At this point, then, we can return to the Kantian definition of life. By virtue of the distinction just outlined, it is clear that, in the eyes of the great German philosopher, the ability to act (*handeln*) in a manner consistent with one's representations is not only human, but extends to all living systems, i.e., to those cognitive systems which, acting for their own benefit, are able to reproduce. Well, this brilliant idea of Kant allows us to reflect on another important issue raised by Kauffman: we are referring to the original idea that the rudiments of semantics, of intentionality, of value and ethics are born with autonomous agents and therefore are intrinsically related to the concept of life. According to the great American scholar, in fact, even if the basics are not enough to leapfrog Hume's naturalistic fallacy, yet with the appearance of autonomous agents the categories of 'ought' and 'is' make their entrance into the physical universe. In this sense, then, self-consciousness, ethics and values could sink their roots in intentionality, a fundamental property of life. In Kauffman's opinion, the rudiment of intentionality is present once an autonomous agent exists. In fact, for the American biologist, ethical behavior first requires the logical possibility of behavior; in virtue of that, one is responsible. In this sense, he argues that to act ethically, someone must be able to act (Kauffman, 2005). In the introduction to the *Doctrine of Virtue*, Kant presents an argument in some ways similar and sometimes surprising, considering his position regarding Hume's law. The great German philosopher expresses himself thus: "[. . .] Conscience is not something that can be acquired, and we have no duty to provide ourselves with one; rather, every man, as an ethical being, *has* a conscience within him originally" (Kant, 1797, p. 400). What does it mean that the root of ethics and of duty resides in being? This expression is used by Kant to break away from the idea that conscience can be acquired. If it could be acquired, it would be something towards which we have a duty: that is, it would be something we do not possess as human beings. To say that every man originally has in himself a conscience does not mean that man is good by nature. This theme is highly topical today: consider, for instance, the neurosciences and in particular the emergence of new areas of research, such as neuroethics.

Some scholars wonder if there are phylogenetically established structures of value that in some way can be linked to chemistry. If the answer to this question is affirmative, man would be that being capable of moral responsibility and whose acts (*that*) could however be considered the result of millions of years of evolution, a result, that is, whose roots would reside in the very capacity of simple autonomous agents to act (*handeln*) to their advantage in their environment (know-how). If so, it would then be possible to infer that man, as the current high point of evolution (if we look at the curve of the brain-size index, *Homo sapiens* represents a real leap), is a sort of linking ring between ethics and biology, i.e., that level of nature in which nature, becoming aware of itself, also becomes a *sine qua non* for the emergence of ethics:

> No man is entirely without moral feeling, for were he completely lacking in susceptibility to it he would be morally dead; and if (to speak in medical terms) the *ethical vital force* could no longer excite this feeling, then humanity would dissolve (by chemical law, as it were) into mere animality and be mixed irretrievably with the mass of other natural beings. But we no more have a special *sense* for what is (ethically) good and evil than for *truth,* although people often speak in this fashion. We have, rather, a *susceptibility* on the part of free choice to be moved by pure practical reason (and by its law), and this is what we call moral feeling" (p. 400).

As is known, for Kant morality is produced by law and not by feeling, however, when speaking of preliminary aesthetic concepts, the German philosopher writes that not to reduce mankind to mere animality we must think of an "ethical vital force" that produces in man a sense that is not a sixth sense because it is not added onto the level at which the other five operate, but is a sort of "morality before morality" whose interface is represented by moral law itself. Given this, in these pages the incompatibilist Kant speaks of the mysterious *ethical vital force* that makes man an ethical vital being. In my opinion, we can glimpse in these words the dawn of a hypothetical theoretical path in which one may hypothesize a naturalistic foundation to the pre-conditions of moral capacity even under the definition of an autonomous agent offered by Kauffman and just now compared with the original Kantian perspective. In this view, then, Boella writes:

> When referring to the scientific and, in this case, neurobiological approach to moral questions, it is appropriate to clarify that this is situated within the context of evolution, but a different question is asked from that of Darwin regarding the natural-biological *origin* of morality, which moreover continues to fuel much debate. Neuroscience can indeed be usefully interrogated in relation to a particular, and certainly not exhaustive, field of the complexity of moral experience, that of the *preconditions or conditions of possibility of moral capacity.* The biological or, more precisely, neurobiological level is therefore *one* level of moral experience corresponding to the existence of automatic reactions, even complex ones, governed by brain mechanisms. This level sets decisive constraints for the exercise of moral capacity and at the same time makes plausible a rooting of moral behavior—for example, altruism, kindness—in the system of desires, intentions, motivations. On the other hand, the multiple ranges of possibilities inscribed in the human brain and its plasticity make it impossible, at least in the present state of knowledge, to attribute even a single moral behavior exclusively to organic functions. In the perspective of human experience in its integrity and richness, it appears that, in every moment of existence, human beings experience the transition from passivity and biological dependence to the realm of judgments, choices, evaluations and actions. And that means that at play are various ways not only of humanizing what is natural, but also of naturalizing what is human" (Boella, 2008, pp. 43–44).

3.5 Awareness, self-organization and intentionality

And here we are inevitably led to the boundaries of neuroethics, that is to say, towards that new field of investigation closely related to the extraordinary progress made in recent years by the brain sciences, and to the entirety of their ethical, legal and social implications. However, these brief references to the interdisciplinary debate underway, regarding the idea of naturalizing ethics and values, show clearly the complexity and scale of these issues. In order, therefore, not to provide answers, but to better frame some of the most important theoretical problems on the table, it is appropriate, at this point of the examination, to continue this work by showing how, in parallel to the research carried out by Kauffman, in recent years in the field of neurobiology a series of studies are cropping up related to intentionality and the biological capacity to choose. In particular, we refer here to W. J. Freeman, an American scholar who, in continuity with Kauffman's perspective, in his 2000 book entitled *How Brains Make Up Their Minds,* shows how intentionality cannot be related only to the level of consciousness but is also present in non-human autonomous agents, and has come to be considered one of the key features of the *bios.* Freeman defines as 'intentional' the brain process in humans and other animals that generates actions aimed at a goal. Typically, such actions are called voluntary if carried out by a human being, but not by an animal because many people think that only humans have the capacity to act by their own will. As an alternative to this concept of volition, therefore, the great neurobiologist attempts to locate a neural basis for purposeful actions which is common to human beings and to other animals, since it reflects the evolution of the human mechanisms from simpler animals in which intention can operate without a will.

The concept of intentionality was first described in 1272 by Thomas Aquinas, who denoted the process by which humans and other animals act in accordance with their own growth and maturation. Therefore we can say that, according to the Italian philosopher, the concept of intent differs both from a motive (reason and explanation of the action) and from desire (awareness and experience stemming from the intent). In Freeman's eyes, physicians and surgeons, differently from philosophers, have preserved the original sense in applying the word 'intention' to the process of growth and healing of the body from injuries (retaining its original biological context). Following this idea, the American neurobiologist sees a profound similarity between the concept of 'intentionality' provided by Aquinas and the term 'assimilation' provided by Piaget: the self comes to understand the world by adapting itself to the world. Thus, the contents of meaning derive from the impact of the world, principally the social impact of actions of other humans upon ourselves, and they include the entire context of history and experience we have already acquired.

Therefore, at the beginning of his book, he expresses himself as follows:

> I believe that animals have awareness, but not awareness of themselves, which is well developed only in humans. Self-awareness is required for volition: animals cannot volunteer. [. . .] I propose that meanings arise as a brain creates intentional behaviors and then changes itself in accordance with the sensory consequences of those behaviors.[. . .] Although the contents of meaning are largely social in origin, the mechanisms of meaning are biological and have to be understood in terms of brain dynamics. Meaning is a kind of living structure [. . .]" (Freeman, 2000a, pp. 8–9).

Neuroscientists have paid little attention to how meaning is born and the conditions that favor it. For pragmatists and existentialists, meaning is clearly shaped by action. In particular, it is created in and by the brain. In Freeman's opinion "meaning is created in unique forms within ourselves through the actions and choices we all make, initially by learning to live according to a system of beliefs offered to us through our parents, peers, or colleagues, first changed to suit ourselves, then modified to become ourselves" (Freeman, 2000a). Usually people assume there is meaning in natural events such as, for example, sunsets, spring flowers and courtship by animals. In reality, the great neurobiologist stresses, meanings are found in the observers (including animals) and not in the objects, events or movements of the body. Only the brain possesses meanings, and these are very different from representations. To fully grasp this difference, then, we must distinguish a mental representation from a state of mind. In Freeman's opinion, the mental content that precedes the execution of an action (mental image) is different from the forms that are frozen into the final result of the action itself (such as a painting or a sculpture). In the American neurobiologist's opinion, this is also true when we compare mental states, thus the investigation should not concern the correlation between a pattern of brain activity with a mental concept in ourselves but, rather, a state of meaning that we infer exists in the brain of the person or other animal that we are observing (Freeman, 2000a).

Today we know much about the anatomical, physical and chemical properties of neurons, but the important thing to understanding fully the relationship between neurons and meaning involves, according to Freeman, a new perspective from which to examine the masses of data collected by neurobiologists and the enigmas arising therefrom. Despite the huge amount of data accumulated, in fact, neuroscientists still are unable to overcome the difficulties posed by the old questions. In this context, the idea of meaning, a critical concept that defines the relationship between each brain and the world, becomes especially fundamental in the debates taking place today in the philosophy of biology, cognitive science, and recently, even neurobiology. As we mentioned before, the process by which meanings are developed and operate is intentionality. For most people, the term *intention* refers to any conscious behavior directed at a target. This sense of the term, as we know, is a diluted version of the concept developed by Thomas Aquinas. Some philosophers of the last century have used the other, mitigated version to describe the relationship (both real and imaginary) between mental states and objects or events in the world. References to this sense of intentionality often talk about the relevance of mental representations.

A major feature of both the everyday and recent philosophical usage of intentionality is an implicit requirement that mental states be conscious. Even though we perform most daily activities that are clearly intentional and meaningful without being explicitly aware of them, as are, for instance, the activities of athletes and dancers, who move themselves in space and time to some end. In fact, taking in consideration the example of sporting activities, we can see that as the training of the brain and body proceeds, the conscious reflection on the manipulation of the body falls away. "Performance becomes 'second nature'" (p. 18).[13] In many cases, the greatest joy and personal fulfillment comes with the individual's total immersion in the activity that disrupts self-awareness: here, individuals become completely one with the object of their desire in body and spirit, without reservation. The brain and the body, anticipating the input signals, perceive and make movements without having to think. It is precisely this kind of ability, unconscious but directed, in the exercise of perception (the know-how, to use Kauffman's and Dennett's term) that the concept of intentionality must include. In light of this, therefore, Freeman reformulates the concept of intentionality on the basis of three fundamental properties: unity, wholeness and purpose. For what concerns unity, we should start by saying that brain and body are entirely committed to the action of projecting ourselves corporeally into the world. Following this idea, we can make a distinction between the self (which is unified) and the awareness of self that we experience as the ego (which is not unified but can be fractured like sunlight on waves). The second property is wholeness: the entirety of life's experience is brought to each moment of action and includes an effort, described centuries ago first by Aristotle and later, by Goethe, as a blind, organic striving toward realizing our full potential within the constraints of heredity and environment. The last property of intentionality is purpose or intent. In this sense we can see that perception is a continuous and mostly unconscious process that is sampled and marked intermittently by awareness. Thus, what we remember are the samples, not the process (Freeman, 2000a). The fact that the description of intentionality does not imply consciousness opens new scenarios. Think, for instance, of the great discoveries made by Owen and colleagues, explained in the first chapter, that are leading us to re-elaborate the traditional relationship between memory, consciousness and intentionality. The possibility to enter into contact through functional magnetic resonance imaging (fMRI) with patients in VS or in a transition state between VS and MCS appears, in fact, to confirm Freeman's theory of meaning, a theory, that is, elaborated since the 80s, and gradually re-defined using more sophisticated models provided by neurodynamics, neurogeometry, the theory of self-organization, the theory of complexity, and the Symbol Dynamic. The distinction between self-consciousness and intentionality and the idea that the self (an integrated synthesis of unity, wholeness and purpose) precedes, also phylogenetically, the emergence of consciousness offers at a philosophical level, an evolutive explanation of the human cognitive processes without diminishing the essential complexity.

The substratum of consciousness, therefore, must be a system composed of many functional different elements which are, however, closely linked together to form an indivisible entity endowed with unity, wholeness and purpose, an entity that has its roots in the infinite bricolage of complex dynamic processes' (internal and external) cutting of new forms in continuous co-evolution.

Evolutionary biologists, in fact, have shown that complex operations of the brain and body have their origin in simpler animals and have evolved into human capacities. In this sense, then, on the basis of data relating to behavior, it is possible to infer that animals harbor intentions, even though we do not know whether they are conscious of their actions. Consider, for example, an animal that wakes up hungry and sets out in search of prey. If it comes across a chemical smell that corresponds to food, it must extract and perceive an odor it is looking for and distinguish it from the whole background of smells, an infinitely complex set of chemicals that it is unable to identify and classify. Then it searches for where the smell is coming from: knowing its origin is part of the smell's meaning. To do this, the animal needs to know where it was when it perceived the smell and calculate its intensity. It must consider several variables, such as wind or water direction, based on the sensation of these on its skin, and on the perception of swaying plants and sounds produced by the current. By virtue of these new inputs, it must continue to move and must know where it has arrived. Finally, it must obtain from sensory receptors in the muscles and joints verification that they have actually done what the brain has told them to do, and if they haven't, it must know what they did instead. Therefore, all of the inputs combined into the unity of a multisensory perception (also known as gestalt) attach to the meaning of the perception (the odor) and none of them to the stimulus (the odorant). Finally, the animal chooses what to do next combining several multisensory perceptions that include its somatosensory records of body movements through its environment (Freeman, 2000a).

The basic activity of searching for food demonstrates the three properties of intentionality identified by Freeman. "Humans evolved from simpler creatures and these earlier forms exhibit precursors of our rich and varied intentional behavior. Evolution has given us the capacity to detect intentionality in others without needing to define it. We recognize directed behavior almost instantly when we see it. [. . .] Charles Darwin found clever evidence for intentional behavior in earthworms, and some scientists believe that even bacteria display it" (p. 30). Consider once again the example of *E. coli* that goes upstream against the glucose gradient in search of food. The "hungry" bacterium distinguishes its own body from external chemical elements, such as a potential food source, and keeps track of its movements in space and time, which may indicate the presence of a wholeness of experience. Its activity is also directed to a specific purpose: reproduction. Naturally, we can only assume all this, by observing the autonomous agent in action. Unity, wholeness and purpose, therefore, are, in the eyes of Freeman, the basic conditions for there to be a biological entity that is a bearer of meaning. As mentioned above, therefore, meanings are transmitted through intentionality, that is, through the process by which living organisms change themselves by acting and learning from the consequences of their actions: when an autonomous agent grasps a meaning, in fact, it is pushed toward new behaviors. Well, depending on the complexity of the autonomous agents, there are different processing capacities for meaning, or different channels of communication. Olfaction remains unique among the senses (for the direct access that its receptor neurons have to the cerebral cortex) and making a comparison of brains, it revealed its important function for the mechanism of intentionality. Therefore, we may observe that visual auditory and somatosensory systems moved in and co-opted the olfactory operating system (the main thrust of dynamics). However, considering the infinite sensory stimuli that the environment gives to the body, we should investigate what are the criteria used by the brain to select what is the stimulus of immediate importance, and what is the biological nature of awareness and how does it work (Freeman, 2000a).

Here we are, therefore, in the presence of one of the great frontiers of the unknown: the appearance and functioning of the human central nervous system, the most deeply teleonomic system that has ever existed on Earth, the only system, that is to say, which generates the mysterious phenomenon of self-consciousness. As Franz Brentano pointed out, inanimate machines do not have consciousness, because they do not have intentions. There is a great deal of debate within the cognitive-science community concerning the nature of consciousness in relationship to artificial intelligence brains and the way it could be considered as the changes of the machine's parts and the behavior of the entire system. In Freeman's opinion these problems are intractable because cognitive science defines meaning as a relation between symbols (in syntactical definitions,, other words and pictures are given in dictionaries), but he further observes that, in reality, references to the world are not defined within a dictionary or computer (Freeman 2000a). Freeman's reflections allow us, at this point, to present the concept of mind offered by pragmatism, a concept that, according to the great neurobiologist, we make our own also in order to shed light on another fundamental aspect of the *bios* that neither Kandel nor even Searle have deepened and that the Kantian definition of life does not grasp in its depth; we are referring here to the fundamental notion of assimilation (or *adaequatio*, a term introduced for the first time by Thomas Aquinas).

For pragmatists, the mind is a dynamic structure derived from actions carried out in the world. Today we know that consciousness interacts with brain processes, yet it is not something epiphenomenal and is not identical to these processes. Consciousness does not control the actions that constitute behavior, at least not directly. In dynamic terms, according to the great neurobiologist, it can be compared to an operator since it modulates the brain dynamics from which past actions have been constructed: "located nowhere and everywhere," it is able to reprocess the contents furnished by the brain's various parts. In humans, according to recent studies, it appears that it is the abundant development of the frontal and temporal lobes that furnishes the object of self-consciousness. Other animals' brains lack these parts and their behavior demonstrates neither self-consciousness nor self-awareness: it is thus possible that they are conscious but not self-conscious, or aware of their intentional actions. When Aquinas was introduced to Aristotle's doctrine of active perception (according to which the organism learns about the world and realizes its potential by its action on the world), he changed this concept, making it conform with Christian doctrine by distinguishing between the will (that makes voluntary ethical choices in regard to good and evil or right and wrong) and intention (the mechanism by which the potential of the organism is realized). In Aquinas' opinion each animal is a unified being enclosed within a boundary that distinguishes the 'self' from the 'other.' In an important passage in the *Summa Theologiae,* the *Doctor Universalis* writes:

> [. . .] to intend is to tend to something; and this belongs to the mover and to the moved. According, therefore, as that which is moved to an end by another is said to intend to the end, thus nature is said to intend to an end, as being moved to its end by God, as the arrow is moved by the archer. And in this way, irrational animals intend an end, inasmuch as they are moved to something by natural instinct. The other way of intending an end belongs to the mover; according as he ordains the movement of something, either his own or another's, to an end. This belongs to reason alone. Wherefore irrational animals do not intend an end in this way, which is to intend properly and principally, as stated above" (Aquinas, 1265–1274, II–II, 12, 5a).

The origin of *understanding* and *intention* is the Latin verb *intendere,* which means not only to strive forward, but also equally important, as we mentioned above, to change oneself by acting and learning from the consequences of one's actions. Instead of Platonic idealism, Thomas sets Aristotelian materialism at the foundation of medieval Church doctrine, though adding a brilliant distinction. Unlike Plato, for Aristotle and Thomas perception is an active process and not a passive acceptance of forms. In the Aristotelian view, however, the interaction between mind and world goes in both directions: transitive actions (for example, cutting, burning, investigating) are directed towards the world as exploratory manipulations, and thus their stimuli enter the body as forms of material objects, while with intransitive actions one interprets and knows the shapes of objects by association. Freeman observes that Aquinas concluded from his conception of the unity of the self that the process is unidirectional. Then, according to Aquinas, we shall see that actions of the body exit by the motor system changing the world and changing the relation of the self to the world. Perception is only the altered contours of the self as experienced inside. The key word that he used is *assimilation* (*adaequatio* means toward, but not at, equality). The body changes its own form to become similar to aspects of stimuli that are relevant to the intent that emerged from within the brain. Aquinas describes this process through the example of something that shines on the inside of a structure, such as a tent. The outside observer infers what is happening from the patterns of reflected light and the movements of the tent walls. Finally, Freeman notes a difference from the walls of Plato's cave, as for Aquinas the forms are created inside the self through achieving similitude and do not come from outside and are imperfectly caught by the senses from the shadows on the passive wall (Freeman, 2000a). Aquinas explains this fundamental concept:

> truth resides primarily in the intellect. Now since everything is true according as it has the form proper to its nature, the intellect, in so far as it is knowing, must be true, so far as it has the likeness of the thing known, this being its form, as knowing. For this reason truth is defined by the conformity of the intellect and thing; and hence to know this conformity is truth. But in no way can sense know truth. For although sight has the likeness of a visible thing, yet it does not know the comparison which exists between the thing seen and that which it itself apprehends concerning it. But the intellect can know its own conformity with the intelligible thing; yet it does not apprehend it by knowing of a thing what a thing is. When, however, it judges that a thing corresponds to the form which it apprehends about that thing, then first it knows and expresses truth. This it does by composing and dividing: for in every proposition it either applies to, or removes from the thing signified by the subject, some form signified by the predicate: and this clearly shows that the sense is true of any thing, as is

> also the intellect, when it knows what a thing is; but it does not thereby know or affirm truth. This is in like manner the case with complex or non-complex words. Truth, therefore, may be in the senses, or in the intellect knowing what a thing is, as in anything that is true; yet not as the thing known in the knower, which is implied by the word truth; for the perfection of the intellect is truth as known. Therefore, properly speaking, truth resides in the intellect composing and dividing (judging); and not in the senses; and not even in the intellect that perceives what a thing is (Aquinas, 1265–1274, I, 16, 2a).

For example, when we adjust one hand to grip a coffee pot and the other to hold a cup in order to fill it, we're not transferring geometric forms in the brain, but uniting our bodies to the forms of the objects, adjusting our hands to manipulate them. Therefore, objects' meanings grow according to what we have done and what we intend to do with them. In this way, others can observe what we are doing, learning by imitation to thereby create meanings similar to ours, though which are produced by them and not transplanted. Thomas based his notion of unidirectionality on the incompatibility between the forms of matter, which are unique and special, and the forms of the intellect, which are generalizations and abstractions. These intellectual constructs are all that we can know because every material object is infinitely complex in its details.

> In one sense truth, whereby all things are true, is one, and in another sense it is not. In proof of which we must consider that when anything is predicated of many things univocally, it is found in each of them according to its proper nature; as animal is found in each species of animal. But when anything is predicated of many things analogically, it is found in only one of them according to its proper nature, and from this one the rest are denominated. So healthiness is predicated of animal, of urine, and of medicine, not that health is only in the animal; but from the health of the animal, medicine is called healthy, in so far as it is the cause of health, and urine is called healthy, in so far as it indicates health. And although healthy is neither in

> medicine nor in urine, yet in either there is something whereby the one causes, and the other indicates health. Now, we have said that truth resides primarily in the intellect; and secondarily in things, according as they are related to the divine intellect. If, therefore, we speak of truth, as it exists in the intellect, according to its proper nature, then are there many truths in many created intellects; and even in one and the same intellect, according to the number of things known (I, 16, 6a).

No two cups are identical, for example, even if they come from the same mold; but for practical reasons, we imagine that they are identical. The forms depend on the size of the objects: in the case, for example, of razor blades, they all look the same to the naked eye; however, when viewed under the electron microscope, each one looks like a different mountain range.

In these circumstances, therefore, Freeman observes that Aquinas dissolved the dichotomy between subject and object. The self creates its unique forms by its assimilation to the world, not by the discovery within itself of ideal forms, categories or eternal truths that are opposed to objects in the world. In other words, the body and the brain are open systems with transmission of matter, energy, and information, but the unidirectionality of perception makes the "fabric of meaning" a closed system. The American biologist further notes that the process of intentionality allows us to take in just as much as we can handle and no more and that perceptional system is our best asset in matching our limited capabilities to the infinite world (Freeman, 2000a). In the doctrine of Thomas Aquinas, as we have shown before, intentionality does not require consciousness, yet it needs action to create meaning. This approach, therefore, allows us to delve further into the theory of the agent as developed by Kauffman. In Freeman's perspective highlighted above, autonomous agents are constructive actors that create ever new meanings through their performance of unpredictable actions (know-how), but this is only possible because, just as Thomas denotes, life is essentially assimilation (*adaequatio*) and thus intentionality: the *bios,* therefore, appears as the result of a transfinite series of adjustments that constitute and modify in unpredictable ways parts of the game itself. We sniff, move our eyes, cup our hands behind our ears and move our fingers to manipulate an object in order to optimize our relationship to that subject for our immediate purpose. Merleau-Ponty calls this dynamic action "search for maximum grip" or "optimization of the relationship of the self with the world done by directing our sensory receptors towards the designated object" (Merleau-Ponty, 1942). Once, after a long and tiring conference, in response to a request to summarize the principle he had devised, the French philosopher said, "To perceive is to be present with respect to something through the body." This sentence contains the main elements of the theme of the conference. Continuing, Merleau-Ponty said, "All the time, the thing keeps its place within the horizon of the world, and the structuring consists in placing every detail within the relevant perceptual horizon" (Merleau-Ponty, 1945). This concept, whether the author intended it or not, is the same as Aquinas' notion of assimilation. Merleau-Ponty seems to draw a distinction between the horizon of the world, outside, and the horizon of perception, inside. In dynamic terms, a person may act on an object and change it, but the object doesn't cross the horizon of their brain, imprinting its own characteristics across the inner horizon of the sensory cortices; you can move toward a horizon, but you can never reach it. If Freeman's interpretation is correct, Merleau-Ponty has grasped the concept of unidirectionality and the solipsistic isolation which suggests the reason why the forms present in matter, according to Thomas, cannot be grasped directly, as all that we can know comes through the imagination. It allows us to generalize and abstract to create the internal structure with which we act and understand. The act of perception transcends the two horizons through assimilation. The structuring is done by repeated cycles of action and perception that Merleau-Ponty calls the intentional arc, which constitutes the effort to achieve maximum grip. In other words, when the French philosopher speaks about his "putting each detail" within the perceptual horizon, he essentially means to position the sensory receptors "efference" and to focus the sensory cortices through "preafference," in order to achieve optimal assimilation of the self to an object (Freeman, 2000a).

Merleau-Ponty's conclusion is that we are moved to action by an imbalance between the self and the world. In dynamic terms, the lack of balance is an endogenous instability that puts the brain on a moving trajectory, that is to say, on a path through a chain of preferred states, which are learned basins of attraction. A nearly final result is not an equilibrium in the chemical sense, which is a dead state, but a descent for a certain period into the basin of an attractor, which gives an awareness of closure. Freeman observes that the aim of phenomenology is to describe sensory experiences without metaphysical preconceptions. But, since phenomenology is the study of the reflection upon and knowledge about phenomena, it is impossible not to involve awareness, as it is the medium through which we experience these constructions and represent them in words. However, Freeman notes at the same time that Merleau-Ponty did refer only occasionally to consciousness, and even less often to awareness, treating consciousness as an epiphenomenon that was unsuitable for scientific study, in contrast with the concreteness of the intentional arc. Freeman disagrees with this vision, as in his opinion science and scientists cannot function without talking and awareness cannot be swept "under the phenomenological rug" (Freeman, 2000a).

In the context of neurodynamics, we think in terms of space and time, thus the question arises whether consciousness is present throughout the intentional arc, or emerges in a segment of the arc and, in this case, in which one. How much time is needed for a journey through the intentional arc and how long after an action or a stimulus has begun does the subject become aware of it? Everyone agrees that this perception takes time. The estimates of the minimum time between noticing the stimulus and learned responses, obtained by measuring the response times of humans and animals, range from one quarter to three quarters of a second. These intervals are longer than the reaction times between painful or pleasurable stimuli and responses that do not require learning, which are less than one tenth of a second.

A similar conclusion was reached by William James, who recounts how one morning, having awoken in his bed, he kept repeating to himself to stand up, to no effect. He stayed under the covers. At one point he found himself standing, unable to remember having gotten up (James, 1890). Merleau-Ponty, too, inferred that consciousness follows action, rather than precedes it. He writes: "It is clear that there is no conceivable causal relationship between the subject and his body, his world and his society" (Merleau-Ponty, 1945, 1964). In Merleau-Ponty's view, therefore, consciousness lies outside the action-perception cycle. "What leads us astray in this regard is that often we look for freedom, free will, in the voluntary decision-making process that examines one reason after another, and seems to opt for that with greater weight, or which is more convincing. In fact, the decision-making follows the decision and it is my secret decision that generates the motives" (Merleau-Ponty, 1945). According to this view, consciousness is not the result of a decision or an effect, but is, according to Searle (but also, in some respects, according to Kandel and Damasio), a relationship between cause and effect, i.e. a mental process. According to Merleau-Ponty's view, actions are not controlled by consciousness because previously, experience creates an interpretation of the present from which action flows without further reflection. Consciousness is unessential to dealing with things intentionally, since most of our daily actions emerge without our thinking about them. But scientific activity is not one of these and phenomenology, in Freeman's opinion, is incomplete unless described with a dynamic process that emerges in the context of neurons and their populations. With this in mind, the question Freeman means to address is how to interpret awareness and consciousness in neurobiological terms. To this end, following the research lines drawn by the American neuroscientist, three premises must first be laid out that constitute a summary of the main points we've developed so far throughout the entire work.

First, the brain is a dynamic system in which each state of consciousness occupies a spatio-temporal synaptic field with configurations of density, impulses and waves and their relative electrochemical components distributed throughout the organ. Each frame occupies a place in a sequence that traverses the space of brain states. This sequence is the trajectory of a state variable, expressing the synaptic residue of past acts of perception and leading to new acts of perception. In such a theoretical framework, consciousness is as much a mental process that we experience phenomenologically as it is a neural process that connects and integrates this sequence of brain states; therefore, it is not just a state variable of the brain. It is also what Freeman, using engineering language, calls an "operator," which mediates operations between neurons. Far from being an epiphenomenon of consciousness, it has to play a crucial role in intentional behavior (Freeman, 1994, 1997, 2004). The task of neurodynamics consists in defining and measuring this role.

Secondly, awareness and consciousness are present in animals with varying content and complexity, corresponding to the variety of structures and brain functions that are found in the animal kingdom. In humans, consciousness takes different forms, due to the complexity of the human brain and human social activity. However, regardless of content, the main operator-state variable should be present in all vertebrates, with the same role of structuring intentional behavior. Freeman believes that it is possible to infer the nature of the operation by analyzing animals' brain dynamics, though we cannot know their contents directly (Freeman 2007, 2009; Damasio, 1994, 1999, 2010).

Third, consciousness can be understood only in the light of a sufficient understanding of causality. Then, according to Freeman we should dwell for a moment on the concept of causality in order to answer some questions regarding, for instance, how reception is caused by actions, and how consciousness is caused by perception. To this end, Freeman affirms, it is necessary to dwell for a moment on the concept of causality. He identifies three meanings of the verb "to cause" which correspond to three different types of causation (Freeman, 2008).

The first meaning is to make, to move, to modulate, and corresponds to Aristotle's efficient cause. The great neurobiologist calls this type of causality "linear causality." Linear causality is what is meant usually when one thinks of causes, in the sense that one always presupposes an agent; think, for example, of the molecular switches identified by Kandel for regulating the transition from short-term to long-term memory and vice versa. When interpreting events according to this conception, each event is assigned a beginning and an end. To demonstrate invariance, one must supply the same stimulus over and over again, and always get the same answer. This procedure, though familiar, is problematic (Freeman, 2008, 2009). The most striking failure of linear causality arises when we study the relationship between microscopic neurons and the macroscopic populations in which they are inserted. Each neuron acts on a myriad of other neurons no more than few synaptic connections away, and the return effect of these neurons already modifies its state before it sends another impulse: hierarchical interaction, therefore, cannot be reduced to a linear causal chain (Freeman, 2000a). These interactions are found not only among the neurons of the neuropil, but also in familiar systems where the particles that make up the ensemble simultaneously create one macroscopic state and are bound by the very same state they have created. The simultaneity violates the requirement that effects follow their cause and the non-linearity of the distributed feedback frustrates any attempt to determine which neurons caused other neurons to fire or not fire. Therefore another type of causality is needed to furnish us with a better description of the relationship between neurons and populations of neurons: "circular causality" (Freeman 2000a, 2000b, 2006).

According to Freeman, the term circular causality, currently widely used by physicists and psychologists, is none other than Aristotle's formal cause, that is, "to explain," "to reason," "to attribute," that is to say, a context in which an explanation is given without invoking an agent. One can appeal to circular causality also to explain the interactions occurring at a higher level between patches and populations of neurons, such as the interaction between the entorhinal cortex and the hippocampus, and, at a still higher level, the interaction found as part of the whole action-perception cycle of the intentional arc, but with a very human touch (Freeman, 1997, 2000b). When we represent such relationships, using words or equations, or geometric or physical models, we make use of a closed ring to describe the activity which flows over time in one direction around the ring (Longo 2012, Petitot, 2008, 2013). Then, in order to understand the ring, according to Freeman, we break the ring into a direct branch and a feedback branch and use linear causality to describe operations in both branches. In other words, we use linear causality, because it describes the subjective experience we have of our own brains' functioning. It is the type of explanation that most humans feel comfortable with (Freeman, 2007). So, we continue to ask in what sense can awareness cause changes in the neural activity that shapes intentional behavior and how, after the suppression of sensory activity, can a newly-structured neural activity cause new awareness (Freeman, Quian Quiroga, 2013).

In order to better frame these issues, attempting thus to come up with some important initial answers, Freeman uses the third meaning of the term "causality," understood as "a human trait that we attribute to objects and events in the world" (Freeman, 2000a, p. 158). This was the conclusion reached by Hume in the eighteenth century, according to which knowledge of causes is only the result of constant conjunctions of events in sequence. It must be said that, four centuries earlier, based on the same premise, Aquinas had come to the same conclusion: the forms in the intellect are created by the imagination and do not lie in the forms taken on by matter (Aquinas, 1265–1274, ch. V.; Freeman, 2000a, p. 159; Basti, 2011). Freeman uses this conclusion to explain the unidirectionality of perception, according to which the forms taken on by the brain's activity in the sensory cortices are created internally and not imposed by the forms of the stimuli. According to this conception, causality is something, the feeling of necessity. It's a threshold in the degree of certainty of prediction that we attribute to a relationship observed in terms of what it portends for our future actions (Freeman, 2000a).

According to Freeman, therefore, keeping complexity theory as a horizon of reference, we can infer that "The action does not need to be accompanied by awareness, but, if it is, we experience the intent to act through preafference of the expected consequences of the act." Thus, we experience our action, or, more precisely, our intention to act, as causing the sensory input, or, more precisely, the constructions that follow the sensory input" (p. 130). Therefore, according to the great neurobiologist, causality is not found in the world outside us, but originates in the neural mechanisms of intentionality from which all knowledge comes. However, on the basis of what has been said so far, we should ask ourselves if it is possible to avoid attributing linear causality and causal action to neurons and populations of neurons. In the past, there have been times when linear thinking has been abandoned, and these precedents may serve as models. The a-causal language of differential equations and tensor calculus, for instance, shifted the old anthropocentric perspective from a focal point on Earth to a new distributed network in the sky. The solar system is held together by the action of gravity, but is structured by the space/time curvature. Today neurodynamics offers precisely this kind of new, broader conceptual framework in which the interactions between the parts that create a whole can be described without recourse to causal agents.

> An elementary example is the self organization of a neural population by its component neurons. The neuropil in each area of cortex contains millions of neurons interacting by synaptic transmission. The density of action is low, diffuse, and widespread. Under the impact of sensory stimulation [. . .] and by the background process of growth and maturation, all the neurons come together and form a mesoscopic pattern of activity. This pattern simultaneously constrains the activities of the neurons that support it. The microscopic activity flows in one direction, upward in the hierarchy, and simultaneously the macroscopic activity flows in the other direction, downward with the arrival of new stimulus [. . .] an entire hemisphere can be destabilized, so it jumps into a new state, and the into another and another, then trading back and forth between the hemispheres in a sequence forming a trajectory (pp. 131–132).

In this view, then, according to Freeman, there must be some form of coordination that explains the unity of intentional action and the tenacity of states directed to a goal despite distractions and unforeseen obstacles. His opinion is that the interactions of neural populations create the global configuration that modulates the amplitude of shared activities in each hemisphere. Populations of neurons are not bound to discharge synchronously, since they retain a high degree of autonomy. Synchronism is detected rarely among individual neurons of a local population. All communities of modules in both hemispheres, which cooperate via the brain stem, the corpus callosum and other inter-hemispheric connectors, express a single global dynamic structure. The micro-macro relationship binding the individual neurons in the populations, then, anticipates the organization of the limbic system and the sensory system in global brain states (Freeman, 2007, 2008; Freeman, Vitiello, 2006, 2008). Once the spatial patterns of global amplitude modulation (AM) have been described and explained, detected by recordings of fields of electrical potentials and magnetic fields inside and on the surface of the cerebral hemispheres, there still remains the task of explaining the relationship with consciousness. In this sense, Freeman notes that the global AM patterns are the biological basis for awareness. He gives the example of how the interactive populations of the brain continually create new local patterns of chaotic activity. The constraint exercised by each module of the brain, acting on others by participating in the global AM pattern, diminishes the freedom of all of them, so the likelihood that anyone of them will destabilize and impose its activity onto other modules is reduced. Freeman finally observes that is really unlikely that any one subset or even a subset of modules could capture the motor systems and shape behavior with minor contributions from other parts (Freeman, 2000a).

The main role played by consciousness, according to this American scholar's original hypothesis, is to prevent precipitous action not by inhibiting, but by extinguishing the local chaotic fluctuations, through a sustained interaction that acts as a global damping constraint, such as what Prigogine describes (1980, 1993). Chaotic fluctuations lead to order, but only those directed toward a basin connected to the intention. The others withdraw continuously, ending in noise, if the order parameter is strong enough (Atlan, 1987; Kauffman, 1993; Freeman, 1994; Nicolis, Prigogine, 1977, 1989). Well, Freeman points out, only a small percentage of the total variance of the activity of each of the modules is embedded in the global configuration, but those small parts are crucial:

> Just as an individual neuron is subject to continual bombardment at its synapses yet can only report out a pulse intermittently on its sole axon, and just as the population is built from the seemingly random activity of millions of neurons yet can form only one attractor pattern at a time, so the whole hemisphere, in achieving unity from its myriad shifting parts, can sustain only one global AM pattern at a time (Freeman, 2000a, p. 135).

Given this, consciousness is a distributed event that integrates the component subsystems and minimizes the likelihood of treacherous state transitions being realized among them. While awareness is a distributed event that integrates the component subsystems and minimizes the likelihood of renegade state transitions in them, consciousness is the process that makes a sequence of global states of awareness. This latter is variable and constrains the chaotic activities of the parts by quenching local fluctuations. In this sense, Freeman observes that consciousness is an order parameter and an operator that comes into play in the action-perception cycle as an action is being concluded and as the learning phase of perception begins. This is one part of the intentional arc in which the consequences of an action that has just been completed are being organized and integrated into meaning and a new action is being developed but is not yet being executed. In other words, consciousness holds back premature action and, by allowing time for maturation and closure, it increases the likelihood of the expression in considered behavior of the long-term premise of an intentional being (Freeman, 2000a). These words allow us to revisit something James wrote in 1879 when struggling with the implications of Darwinian natural selection for brain activity. In an article titled, "Are we automata?" the great scholar wondered whether consciousness could have a functional role, giving its owner a competitive advantage. The contrary view regarded consciousness as an epiphenomenon that can allow us to know God and experience pleasure or pain, without affecting the activity of the neurons that produce it. James concluded that consciousness is an "organ added in order to govern a nervous system grown too complex to regulate itself" (James, 1879). But, in Freeman's opinion it is not an organ in the sense of some part of a brain. It is, rather, a higher level of self-organization (Freeman, 2000a).

Interesting here is the holistic perspective: in the interpretation of consciousness as a dynamic operator capable of creating order, there suddenly appears a purpose (an ordered totality) that is incompatible with any vitalistic theory and which, however, turns out to be regulated by a mysterious dual game of constraints (invariance) and possibilities (the becoming of multiplicity). The idea of organization, of wholeness, then, in itself demands a purpose insofar as it is not possible to separate the structure from its meaning. Freeman, therefore, closely joining Prigogine's theory of dissipative structures and H. Maturana and F. Varela's study of autopoietic systems, as well as studies of cybernetics, molecular biology, biomathematics, bioinformatics, Kandel's biology of memory and functional semantics, initiates a process of widening the articulation of complexity theory by showing how such a theory no longer refers only to the simple survey of phenomena, of a dissipative character of a Markovian mold, but extends to consider also the phenomena of transformation of information as well as how such phenomena are generated from the constitution of a biological system for processing information itself. Natural systems, in fact, as affirmed by Atlan (2000) and Carsetti (2000a), are characterized by the fact that what self-organizes within them is the very function that determines them and their meaning. In the light of these considerations, the study of brain functions is the real key to scientific investigation within the complexity of natural (biological) systems. According to this perspective, information is not found in specific and determinable places; on the contrary, the system acts as a dynamic whole within which each particular becomes indispensable when it enters into interaction with the others, giving birth, thus, to a complex self-organization. Behold the emergence, therefore, of the fundamental notion of distributed programs. If we want to maintain the metaphor of the calculator, as Freeman does, we could describe consciousness by using the mechanical metaphors of the thermostat which samples and adjusts the temperature, in which programs (or networks) and data are distributed parallel to one another on a global level. In this case, the data's and program's respective roles are related: what counts as data in a program is often the product of a second program, and the product of the first program often serves as data for a third or for the very first program that has provided the initial data. The phenomena of consciousness and memory, therefore, are related not only to a program inscribed in the double helix, but to a series of distributed programs joined to self-programming functions: it is precisely this that constitutes the notion of biological meaning. The authentic information of the *bios* is not in bits (it does not correspond to simple binary logic), but rather should be sought in the semantic field: it corresponds to the logic of chance, that is, to that logic proper to living beings (Atlan, Louzoun, 2007; Atlan, 1998, 2000; Carsetti, 1999, 2004, 2005b; Kauffman *et al.*, 2008; Di Bernardo 2011). However, while Prigogine and Kauffman[14] mostly use Boolean mathematical models (Boolean stochastic networks) to interpret the mind, Freeman and above all, as we shall see shortly, Atlan and Carsetti attempt to go beyond this logic of reference, also going in new directions. Atlan, in this perspective, in his 1985 article entitled "Complexity disorder and self creation of meaning" thus writes:

> "In very general terms, what characterizes self-organization is an optimal state that lies between the two extremes of a rigid, immovable order, unable to change without being destroyed, like the order of a crystal, and a constant renewal and without any stability, a renewal that evokes chaos and smoke rings. Evidently this intermediate state is not fixed, but allows the being to respond to random, unforeseen perturbations, through organizational changes that are not a simple destruction of the pre-existing organization, but rather a reorganization that allows new properties to emerge. These new properties can be a new structure, or a new behavior influenced in turn by new structures: and the structures or behaviors are new in the sense that, *a priori*, nothing allowed us to foresee them in their details and specificity (p. 142).

Based on these considerations it is clear that, since the eighties, the birth of complexity theory has favored, in the eyes of the scientific community, the emergence of a new concept: self-programming. Still today, this concept constitutes the fundamental property characterizing every living organism. In the dynamics of self-organization, in fact, it is the very functioning of the entire brain and body that creates genetic information: meaning is not added, but, on the contrary, generates the syntax (the sequence of nucleotide bases at the level of the genome and the synaptic connections in the brain) (Carsetti, 2007, 2009a, 2009b; Atlan, 2011; Freeman, Vitiello 2009; Di Bernardo 2012).

According to this perspective, then, the biological meaning, the "hidden face" of genetic information (at the cellular level) and brain information (at the level of neuron populations), represents that creative and organizing function that, immersed in time, is the basis of life, memory and consciousness. Organisms manipulate themselves and perform, therefore, to the extent that their system constitutes itself as an autonomous reality; the origin of the meaning of the system's self-programming reveals itself, objectively, as an emergent property. In this sense, then, in agreement with Atlan and Carsetti, we can summarize what we mean by self-organization by stating that "self-organization means allowing chance to acquire a meaning, *a posteriori*, in a given context of observation" (Carsetti, 1984, 2000a, 2000b; Atlan, 2000). In other words, this means that the complexity of a structure or behavior, which may appear as an irreducible uncertainty, can be eliminated by using another kind of randomness when it becomes possible to observe how that uncertainty causes new meanings to emerge. "This, in our opinion, is the consequence of the close relationship that exists between complexity and chaos in natural systems (not planned by man). The only difference between complexity and disorder is, in fact, the existence or non-existence of a function that is meaningful in the eyes of the observer" (Atlan, 1985, p. 149).

According to Freeman, then, the biology of meaning includes the whole brain and the body, with the personal history that incorporates the experience in the bones, muscles, endocrine glands and neural connections. A state endowed with meaning, according to the great neurobiologist, is a configuration of activities of the nervous system and of the body that has a particular focal point in the space of the organism's states, not in the physical space of the brain.

> The elements of each dynamic state consist of the pulses and waves in the brain, the contractions of the muscles, the joint angles of the skeletal system, and the secretions of cells in the autonomic and neuroendocrine systems. Meanings emerge from the whole of the synaptic connections among the neurons of the neuropil, the sensitivities of their trigger zones, determined by the neuromodulators, and to lesser extents the growth, form, and adaptations of the rest of the body" (Freeman, 2000a, p. 115).

Therefore, in accordance with brilliant insights advanced by the great neurobiologist, we can infer that every human person is

> a 'source of meaning,' a perennial source for the flow of new constructions circulating in the brain and body, protected by the secrecy of isolation. Our constructions are, in fact, due

> to the luxuriant growth of configurations of neural activity arising from the chaotic dynamics of populations composed of myriads of neurons. Our intentional actions pour themselves continuously into the world, changing the world itself and the relationship between our body and external reality. This dynamic system is the self in each of us. The perception of the world from inside changes ourselves by assimilation. Our actions are considered as a realization of an inner *telos* known by representations (Freeman, 2000a).

This being the case, then, how do we perceive the self? Is there, perhaps, something more than memories of experiences gathered into the unity of intentionality? Self-consciousness, according to Freeman, implies, as we have seen, a further level of organization above that of consciousness, a level that only exists in humans and to a very limited extent in some of our closest relatives: the great apes. The difference in the organization of the space of brain states must be in some way related to the difference found in the organization of the brain's anatomy between ourselves and animals who are very different from us. The best place to start are the differences in relationships between the limbic system and the vast areas of the frontal and temporal lobes that have been added to the human brain over the last half million years of evolution (Freeman, 2000a, 2000b).[15]

From these considerations, therefore, in my opinion it is possible to infer that life is not just language (or at most, a pure system of programs) and cognition (and, in general, learning), but also appears as a co-evolutionary phenomenon where information is continuously transformed giving birth, moreover, to a dialectical process of creation and assimilation (*adaequatio*) of ever new meanings: behold thus, for Freeman, Atlan and Carsetti, the emergence of an unpredictable phenomenon, that is, a complexity that emerges from chaos and that proves to be endowed with intentionality. Hence the need on the part of contemporary complexity theory to identify increasingly sophisticated tools designed to account for the origin of living forms and their self-organization. These tools would help identify elements for the elaboration of a theory able to address the intentional complexity of life, exploring the possibilities of building a new process semantics that can be applied to biology; i.e., a semantics that is no longer just of the interpretative kind, but rather of the generative kind (Carsetti, 1999). In recent years, the request has come from various parts of the world to define the principles of a new algorithmic information theory, not exclusively anchored to a propositional base, but articulated at the level of a dimension of a predicative and stratified logic.[16]

3.6 Memory, visual cognition and meaningful complexity

As we have amply shown in the previous paragraphs, by applying to cognitive study the theories of complex nonlinear systems, the biology of memory, the methods introduced by neurodynamics and brain imaging techniques, researchers are slowly coming to discover precise answers to a whole series of questions that have always animated philosophical debate and debates in cognitive science, and are delineating guidelines for what concerns a scientific examination of the issues involved in the mind, intentionality and consciousness. In fact, thanks to the results obtained from basic research in the fields of molecular biology and cognitive science, and by virtue of their integration into a broader theoretical framework capable of holding together the approach linked to methodological reductionism, the informational approach and the holistic one, that is to say, the proper domain of complexity theory in its widest articulation, scientists are beginning to find, as we have just seen, univocal and unambiguous answers to relevant questions such as: what brain processes constitute and "represent" the mnestic and perceptual activity as a whole? How can we define the relationship between mind and brain? How can we explain the nature of direct and primary perceptual processes when we know that at the level of the underlying nonlinear dynamics, there are a multitude of competing mechanisms? What tools and mathematical modeling we can use to define their processes of self-organization, as they occur at the level of perception and cognition? And moreover, what explanation can we give to the relationship that exists between the assimilation of emerging "qualities," on the one hand, and adaptive processes, on the other? Finally, what is the profound link between meaning and knowledge building?

Indeed, current models of cognition based on nonlinear dynamical systems are not yet able to offer an adequate explanation of the ultimate reality of perception and memory, phenomena characterized by recondite forms of continuous emergence, and by the ability to go beyond the surface appearance of things, to arrive at their profound significance, to capture, that is, what we might associate with Frege's *Sinn* (Frege, 1892) or even Husserl's concepts of "substrate" and "organicity" (Husserl, 1939, 1952a, 1952b). In other words, it is necessary to presuppose that the brain's level of sophistication and complexity is significantly greater than that of the Boolean networks used by connectionists, capable of propositional classifications, such as, for example, the Hopfield networks (1982), but lacking a polyadic and intentional dimension.

From an epistemological point of view, cognition can be characterized in terms of an effective response to a difficult question: "How is information assimilated?" Concerning this question, in agreement with Carsetti, we must understand that,

> the assimilation process of external information implies the existence of specific forms of determination at the neural level as well as the continuous development of a specific cognitive synthesis. Actually, information relative to the system stimulus is not a simple amount of neutral sense data to be ordered, it is linked to the unfolding of the selective action proper to the optical sieve, it articulates through the imposition of a whole web of constraints possibly determining alternative channels at, for example, the level of internal trajectories (Carsetti, 2009a, p. 283).

The process of assimilating external information implies the existence of specific defining forms at the neural level. Depth information, moreover, engages in recurrent cycles of self-organizing activity, characterized by the formation of continuous attractors arranged on a variety of levels:

> If I manage to close each time the 'garland' successfully, and imprison the thread of meaning, thereby harmonizing with

> the ongoing 'multiplication' of mental processes at the visual level, I posit myself as an adequate grid-instrument for the progressive and coherent 'surfacing' of depth information and for its self-generating and unfolding as *Natura Naturata,* a Nature which the very units (monads) of multiplication will then be able to read and see as such (i.e. as a great book—library—of natural forms written in mathematical characters) through the eyes of mind (Carsetti, 2004, p. 311).

The cognitive processes insofar as they are characterized by procedures of self-organization are based, therefore, in accordance with Carsetti, on the gradual building of a "subject-I" characterized by a progressive work of abstraction, unification and emergence that leads, on the one hand, to the partial creation and interpretation of external reality and, on the other, to the establishment of that same subject as cognitive subject. A subject, that is, able to descend into the bowels of society, nature and history, and that, through a real biological transformation, driven by knowledge, may finally result in the emergence of a profound evolutionary revolution. In other words, the brain's role appears to be that of providing a self-organizing measurement space of an essentially biological nature. Such an apparatus would be developed, by necessity and in a progressive manner, through a set of processing stages characterized by continuous patterns of interaction and integration:

> This priming property emphasizes that the visual cortex is not merely a feed forward filter that passively detects visual features, as was proposed by many scientists who thought of the visual brain [. . .] as a feed forward hierarchy of bottom-up connections that form increasingly complex and large-scale receptive fields. Rather, the visual brain is an integrated system of bottom-up, top-down, and horizontal interactions which actively completes boundary groupings and fills in surface representations as its emergent perceptual units. This interactive perspective has enabled recent neural models to quantitatively simulate the dynamics of individual cortical cells in laminar cortical circuits. Such results represent a concrete proposal for beginning to solve the classical Mind/

> Body Problem, and begin to do justice to the exquisite sensitivity of our visual percepts to the scenes and images through which we know the visual world (Grossberg, 2004, pp. 29–30).

In these circumstances, therefore, if you want to build appropriate formal models of cognition you must necessarily develop and explore "autopoietic models" able to interact with the same dynamic aspects they intend to describe. These models will have a self-referential capacity of representation able to allow, through their own metamorphosis, for a Nature that is always new, expressing itself according to its deepest dimension. As we have stated several times already, cognition is not only a process of self-organization, it is also the end result of a coupled process of cooperation and synthesis. If we consider, therefore, the external environment as a complex, multiple and layered source, in interaction with the nervous system, we can easily understand, as in fact Carsetti (2004) has noted, how cognitive activities, dedicated to the intelligent search for depth information, could lead to a change in the same conditions through which the Source progressively expresses its own action. In this sense, the simulation models are neither neutral nor purely speculative. Real knowledge appears to be necessarily connected to exact forms of reading, which allow a specific and coherent deployment of depth information contained in the Source. In other words, the simulation models of cognition, to be valid, must show themselves to be creative channels, autonomous functional systems, the very roots of a possible development of the entire system represented by the mind and its reality (Carsetti, 2006). Cognitive activity is, therefore, rooted in reality, but at the same time represents the necessary means through which reality itself can become embodied in an objective way, that is to say, through which it can incorporate itself according to a process of deep nesting and surface deployment of the operative meaning. In this sense, according to Carsetti, it is possible to say that the objectivity of reality is also a measure of the autonomy achieved by the procedures of cognition. The procedures of reference, in this sense, play a guiding role, one of reflection, analysis and channeling of the primary information flows and the selective forces at play. At the same time, these are at the basis of the operations of the "imprisonment of meaning" and "registration of the file as self-generative system" (Carsetti, 2005a).

In light of all this, therefore, cognition appears as the final result of a construction performed under the conditions of experience. It is "live" and organic because it is not the product of simple mental associations that can be reviewed; to the contrary, it arises as the harmonious and targeted articulation of specific attractors according to different levels of implication.

> The resulting texture is experienced on a conscious level by means of self-reflection: we feel, in fact, that it cannot be reduced to anything else and that it proves to be, rather, primary and self-constituting. Taking hold of information at the visual level means 'capturing' and 'playing' each time, in an inner generative language, through progressive assimilation, selection and real metamorphosis and according to 'genealogical' modules, the articulation of the complex semantic apparatus which works at the deep level and molds and subtends, in a mediate way, the presentation of the functional patterns at the level of the optical sieve" (Carsetti, 2012a, p. 17).

The model can delineate itself as such and manage, thus, to open the eyes of the mind to the extent that it is able to allow the categorial to anchor itself to intuition. It is precisely in relation to the proper creation of the channel that a sieve can effectively articulate itself and perform, in this way, its own selective work on an informational level.

> It is exactly through a similar self-organizing process, characterized by the presence of a double selection mechanism, that the mind can partially manage to perceive (and assimilate) depth information in an objective way. The extent to which the network model succeeds, albeit partially, in encapsulating the secret cipher of this articulation through a specific chain of programs determines the model's ability to see with the eyes of the mind. To assimilate and see, the system must first 'think' internally [. . .] the secret structures of the possible

> and, then posit itself as a channel [. . .] for the process of opening and of deployment of depth information (Carsetti, 2009a, pp. 284–285).

Thus, the memory as emergence, as continuous process of opening up of depth information (generated by the complex dialectics between vision, thought and external world) means grasping the routes and modalities that determine the selective and coupled action expressed by meaning, that is, the modalities related to the semantic apparatus' revealing itself on a surface level. In this sense, if we wish to explain how the mnestic process is articulated according to the principles of the theory of self-organization, we must, of necessity, combine the measures regarding semantic information (and not just statistical rarity), on the one hand, and measures concerning computational incompressibility, on the other. We must, in particular, define and implement measures capable of taking into account the coupled connection between the Source and the cognitive agent, the evolution of this same connection, as well as the later creation of meaning as its symbolic form (Atlan, 2000). Only in this way will it be possible to understand how a natural cognitive system may come to be articulated as a system of observation and learning and, simultaneously, as a "self-organizing measuring tool in the world and of the world" (Carsetti, 2008). At the level of meaningful memory of living systems, the selection made by meaning becomes autonomous primarily to the extent that it proves capable of coherently "modulating" the continuous eruption of "new generative systems that characterizes the existence of the original Source" (Carsetti, 2013). Thus, in Carsetti's opinion, it is revealing itself as autonomous in the invention of a new possible incompressibility that, in effect, determines the emergence of a new creativity, also through the narration of its "work-construction":

> [. . .] at the level of a biological cognitive system sensibility is not a simple interface between absolute Chance and an invariant intellectual order. On the contrary, the reference procedures, if successful, are able to modulate canalization and create the basis for the appearance of ever new frames of incompressibility through morphogenesis. [. . .] These

> procedures are in actual fact functional to the construction and irruption of new incompressibility: meaning, as *Forma formans*, offers the possibility of creating a holistic anchorage, and it is exactly what allows the categorial apparatus to emerge and act according to a coherent 'arborization' (Carsetti, 2012a, p. 22).

It is in this way, according to the Italian scholar, that one can ensure that there is a time of invention, a time, namely, of the renewal and discovery that are continually revealed as possible in proportion to the work. The new incompressibility that is born determines each time the selection in place. To do this, the procedures of reference must act as an arch between invariance (the maximum of the potential variability), on the one hand, and autonomous morphogenesis, on the other (Carsetti, 2008). I can, therefore, come to see the principles for a new incompressibility that comes to manifest itself, through the mnestic process, as the fusion of emerging nuclei of creativity in the unity of the "operant meaning." The new invention that is born then gives rise to the emergence and opening of new eyes of the mind: "I see as a mind because new meaning is able to articulate and take root through me" (Carsetti, 2012a, p. 22). Such rooting, however, is based, in turn, on the emergence that occurs at the informational level.

Memory, therefore, according to what has been said so far, is not simple recognition or a simple replication. It can be interpreted, first of all, as a reading-execution of the unity in the making of the original body of meaning with operant self-organization and at human level self-reflection. At this point in the analysis, therefore, in the context of contemporary complexity theory and in particular at the level of the lines of research that in these last few years have come to prioritize the study, at the level of non-standard models, of the complex relationship between perception and thought, we may attempt to develop a parallel between vision and memory, there where memory comes to configure itself on both the epistemological and the phenomenological level as a process of continual representation and reorganization of depth information where each lived moment is presented to consciousness as an integrated whole, a dense flow of images, that is to say, as a clear cut telos which, while respecting certain constraints, comes to unfold itself before the eyes of the mind as vision, a "vision" which by principles is progressively identifying itself as "I" and brain in action, as a Cogito characterized by an objective (neural) existence. Therefore, following the research lines traced in these last few years by Freeman, Grossberg, Petitot and especially Carsetti, in my opinion, remaining within the horizon of epistemological research, it is legitimate to ascribe to memory what is true of vision. This involves, namely, a process of progressive identification and assimilation of unity in terms of an adequate plot of self-organizing programs "able to portray itself as such, a process which becomes gradually autonomous and through which, via selection, in a renewed way and at the surface level, Reality can canalize the primary modules of its own complex creative tissue: i.e. surfacing as generativity and nesting as meaning" (Carsetti, 2009a, p. 297). The original creativity that surfaces and the emerging meaning blend, thus, in the expression of a "work" that comes, finally, to be articulated in a consistent manner within itself and to fuse itself with the I-subject as synthesis (by images) and narration in act: an observer can, therefore, come to identify itself through the work's development as a "watermark" (Carsetti, 2013). The resulting pathway is capable of ensuring, in this way, a real conjunction of function and meaning. In such a framework, the notion of complexity, according to Carsetti, therefore expresses interpersonal skills, functional coordination, interdependence, ways of generating articulated processes in which different parts must work together and do so in a fitting way. Here complexity is not complication or unpredictability, but generativity in action, that is, the process of opening and deployment of depth information (meaningful complexity), a process, that is to say, whose result is given not by generative principles, but by self-organizing forms in action. Hence the possibility of considering nature (and therefore consciousness and memory as its processes and/or properties) at the same time as emergence, as depth information hiding itself through the emergence of ever new postulates of meaning; this emergence will be matched by the progressive appearance of ever new constraints (forms and rules) at the generative level. According to this concept of complexity, therefore, life is articulated each time through the "identification-reading" of that particular and coordinated series of "functional closures," of that specific chain of "fixed points"[17] that is required for the coherent deployment of the source along the paths of invariance and in accordance with "its original creativity"(Carsetti, 2008). In this sense, at the level of the emergence and self-reflection in action, the adequate work of unification-closure of the network's own programs, which encapsulates the selection made internally by meaning, constitutes the real basis of memory and cognition. In fact it comprises a plurality of interconnected works, each of which is connected to a consciousness. In this way, the above unification necessarily concerns the continuous interweaving of a unitary consciousness, though within the original fragmentation of micro-consciousnesses and of the divided self (Carsetti, 2009b, 2012b) in agreement with Freeman's intentionality theory and with the non-standard approaches elaborated, in an independent way, by Damasio (who distinguishes at the phylogenetic level the appearance of the self from that of the mind) and by Zeki, father of the concept of micro-consciousness. These approaches have in common with the non-standard models, here delineated, the key concept of the disunified self on the basis of the existence in natural systems of micro-cognitive units interconnected as a kind of virtual web in continuous growth (Zeki 1999; Damasio 2010; Freeman, 2000a, 2000b).

It is according to this point of view that memory, as well as cognition, appears necessarily related to a process of continuous emergence, in turn connected to the progressive articulation of a self-organizing and self-expressing I. To the extent that the system manages to remember, it emerges toward itself and can, therefore, identify and narrate (above all through images) itself as an "I" and, specifically, as an I that sees and grasps the meaning of things with particular regard to the meaning linked to the emergence concerning them. In the moment in which the aforementioned work becomes vision, according to Carsetti, it simultaneously reveals itself as construction in act and at the same time as the filter and the connecting thread of a cohesive canalization through which new reality can come to reveal itself in the unfolding of its own deep creativity (Carsetti, 2006). Meaning-rich forms will, therefore, come into play, they will be reflected in a work and will come to be seen by an I that can thus build itself revealing itself as real autonomy (cognition in act and intentionality). "The I-subject will recognize itself through the coordinated action of these observation systems; it will mirror itself in the 'pupils' of these very systems to the extent that it will be recognized as the primary factor of their recovery as autonomous units" (Carsetti, 2004, p. 325). In this sense, "nature is the very (original) opening of the process of determination. It presents itself as a dynamic system of meaningful processes in action; the 'method' in its turn must offer real instruments in order to feed and coagulate the self-organizing growth and the articulated unfolding of these very processes. On the other hand, Nature must also be considered as a body-system of meaning that cannot be occupied" (p. 326). In the light of the understanding achieved so far by following the path laid out by some relevant research by Carsetti about the concept of the fixed point, in my opinion it seems possible to affirm that the inner world as perceived by virtue of complex mnestic processes is constituted not of static forms, but of processes that seem full of meaning; processes, namely, that, from a biological and functional point of view, can be considered as acting information + intentionality. Just as the meaning of words is connected with a universe of highly dynamic functions and functional processes that effect combinations, deletions, additions (a universe that, according to Carsetti, we can only describe in terms of symbolic dynamics), in the same way, at the level of the memory, similar patterns are continually being revealed and built and made available for the selection offered by coordinated information penetrating from external reality (Carsetti, 1999, 2004, 2013). All this ultimately comes to intertwine with "the mechanisms of internal selection during a 'journey' in the regions of intentionality" (Carsetti, 2012b).

Memory, in this sense, in my opinion, is the process of inscription, reconstruction, assimilation and reduction that occurs through a dual selection and in accordance with the precise dialectic process between form and information by which forms in action inhabit life. At this level we see that in a natural autopoietic system, what is truly self-organizing is the function together with its meaning. In the case, for example, of natural language the origin of meaning in the complex organization of the system is nothing more than an emergent property. Husserl (1908) would say that "meaning has the power to produce forms." Grammar then ultimately reveals itself as the grammar of thought, of a thinking that cannot be distinguished from language in action, from a language that gradually constitutes itself as "the very word of reality" (Husserl, 1931, 1952b). The processes of emergent computation, therefore, as we have seen, prove to be linked to the arising of a precise non-linear symbolic dynamic.

Complexity theory, as prefigured according to a purely epistemological point of view, comes gradually to emerge as a complex system of rules, constraints and references that stretches on forever. Within this game one of the basic problems that seems to emerge is that already outlined by Thomas Aquinas in his small work *De Principio Individuationis.* The problematic reality of a person's life is seen today in the light of current awareness as a genetically determined reality, a reality that goes from conception to the progressive formation of the neural structures, structures that live thanks to precise biochemical processes characterized by highly complex forms. This long journey leads to the identification of a unique entity, different from all the others, capable of conceiving the world that surrounds it in a totally unique manner. Maximum complexity thus comes to coincide with maximum "individuation." The most general reading and modeling instruments should be used, therefore, to understand the most singular and individual reality that exists on earth. So next to the concepts of complexity, choice, and process, a concept at once new and old comes to take shape: the concept of person (Tonini, 1983; Del Re, 2000). Alongside the epistemology systems, therefore, a new type of knowledge arises on the horizon: an anthropology[18]. Thus, complexity theory enables us to pass from a theory of information that elaborates signs to an anthropology that sees in the naturalization of cognitive processes not the threat of materialism, but the opportunity to elevate the biological to a meta-level. Saying that consciousness is a natural process (Searle, 2004, 2007; Carsetti, 2008, 2009a, Damasio, 2010) is not to reduce it to simple molecular mechanisms or to a solely material reality. Current scientific research shows that matter can give rise to extraordinary properties; indeed, it can be held that matter itself is derived from complex processes of energy exchange (force fields), from processes, that is, already shaped by a form. The central thesis of this book, therefore, is that consciousness and memory are highly complex processes that depend on the particular dispositions of matter, though not being reducible to it[19] (Siegel, 1999; Freeman, 2000a; Searle 1997; Edelman, 2004, 2006).

In the case of the human being we are dealing with a single subject that is, so to speak, scanned according to many levels of intelligibility which, however, must be geared towards unity. If we were to account for that object through only one of these levels, we would wrong not only the object, but also the discipline attempting to offer a complete explanation of it, since the object we are trying to understand is complex, that is, not reducible to being studied under a single approach. Consider, for example, the multiplicity of levels on which man can be explained, where the latter can be considered as: the unity of his chemical and physical components (carbon chemistry and its properties), the unity of his genetic patrimony and of his belonging to a species (genetics, zoology, paleoanthropology), the unity of his biological processes (biology and physiology), led by the unity of his being an individual, as revealed, for example, in the functions of feeding, homeostasis, self-healing and reproduction (philosophy of life), the unity of consciousness and of self-awareness (Tanzella-Nitti, 2012a, 2012b). To arrive, finally, at a higher form of unity, the form of a self-conscious personal I guided in its actions by an inner light, a light, that is to say, that reveals itself to consciousness as free will.

In this spirit, therefore, we will continue our analysis by first hearing the authoritative voice of Daniel J. Siegel, the father of neurobiology of intersubjectivity, currently director of the Infant and Preschool Service at the University of California and professor of psychiatry at the UCLA School of Medicine, who by integrating Kandel's biology of memory, Prigogine's theory of dissipative structures, neurobiology, neurodynamics and neuroimaging techniques, as well as complexity theory, psychological research and cognitive science, and starting from the assumption that brain structure and function are formed directly by interpersonal experience, furnishes new answers regarding the formation of sense of self, that is, how the encounter between our brains and our experience makes us who we are.

Chapter 4

Sense of Self: A Non-standard Approach

4.1 Interpersonal connections, auto-regulation and integration

As demonstrated in the previous chapters, from the eighties onwards research in neuroscience developed rapidly, moving in the direction of ever greater connection between biology and the psyche. The Nobel Prize winner Eric Kandel (2000), as we have seen, contends that the new advances in neurobiology and psychiatry have permitted an important cross fertilization between the two fields, removing the prejudices and acts of faith of the respective schools of thought. In particular it has permitted psychoanalytical insights to direct research on the deeper understanding of the neurobiological bases of behavior. Thus, the theories of the psychic perspective and the somatic perspective acquire scientific legitimacy that are born simultaneously in and of the link. It clearly emerges that the development of the nervous system is an "experience dependent" process: in the first phases of life significant relationships are indeed the primary source of experiences and even modulate genetic expression at the level of the brain. Relationships with others have a fundamental influence on the brain: the circuits that mediate social experiences are tightly correlated with those responsible for integration of the processes that govern attribution of meaning, the organization of memory as well as the modulation of emotional responses and the regulation of the functions of the organism. Research in the realm of neuroscience and genetics, therefore, is opening new scenarios now where, on the one hand there is the opportunity to rediscover the unsurpassable limit that both distinguishes and unites the body with the mind, feeling with self-awareness, on the other the question is being posed regarding the crucial role that neurophysiological mechanisms and genetic predisposition have in determining behavior, thoughts and actions. Daniel J. Siegel in *The Developing Mind* (1999) studies the mind as a product of the interactions between interpersonal experiences and structure and functions of the brain, incorporating knowledge that comes from neurobiology, psychological research and cognitive science and an intense clinical activity carried out on children and their parents. Taking into consideration the research done by Squire and Kandel (2009) Siegel examines the grave consequence that unintegrated approaches have both for the study of the brain and the mind noting how the interactions with the environment and in particular relations with others have a direct influence on the development and structures of the brain, therefore, the unintegrated approach can be counterproductive in the attempt to understand the development of the human mind (Siegel, 1999).

Moreover, Siegel analyses the mechanisms with which social and relational factors mold the development of the brain and mind, favoring the achievement of an emotional equilibrium. He examines subjective and relational experiences as well as ordinary and pathological ones with reference to the nature of the processes through which our brain perceives other minds and the ways in which brain circuits develop, after birth, in the presence of emotional status depending on relationships with others and with the external world. He focuses his theoretical proposal on three levels: the first is the neurobiological level, which analyses neuronal activity in terms of flow, energy consumption and continuously evolving networks (nervous connections); the second one sees the mind as a processor of information that allows the reception of sensory stimuli coming from the environment and their representation in the form of patterns of neuronal excitement corresponding with mental symbols, and that places bodily sensations and perceptions mediated by the five senses in direct connection with ideas, concepts and words; finally, the last level is that of interpersonal relations and the relationships that characterize the first years of life and that can facilitate or inhibit this tendency to integrate the representation of various experiences, directly influencing the capacity for mental reconstruction of reality (Sbattella, 2006). Siegel's thesis can be summarized as follows: "Human connections form the development of the nervous connections that form the mind" (Siegel, 1999, p. 4) and at the center of the reciprocal influence between experiences and evolution of brain structure and functions are the processes of communication and organization of the emotions, as well as the processes of integration that the mind operates to produce coherence between the different states of the self. In Siegel's opinion integration is a process (and not a final accomplishment), defined as the mutually influencing interactions between two or more relatively independent and differentiated entities. Thus, integration allows for the spontaneous flow of energy and information within the whole brain, and this is the flexible influence of layers of processes upon each other. In his volume and in many articles Siegel insists on the plasticity of the complex structures and human cerebral connections, typically sensitive, even in old age, to the game of forces activated by the exercise of memory, by emotional experience and by phenomena of attachment. This sensitivity, which is only partly determined by the inherited genetic baggage, is strongly conditioned by the processing an individual is capable of performing in terms of containing and modulating the affective and relational sphere of his or her lived experience. Fundamentally, it is the capacity to organize one's experience along the axis of a temporal sequence endowed with meaning.

Siegel, therefore, does not propose merely a critical review of some paths to support the direction of a contamination that moves in the direction that is unique to a psychiatry influenced by neuroscience, but offers a systemic approach, able to go beyond the mere differentiation of specialised knowledge and at the same time to hold together procedures and principles. The specificity of the disciplines and the complex language of each area of study must be placed in a work of analysis and translation that may finally lead to a synthesis based on continuous dialogue between different and complementary types of knowledge. One example is the concept of *integration* which, next to that of plasticity, manages to give an account of a wider identity, although not all carried out under the sign of conscious rationality. The idea of integration proper to an adequate epistemology allows one to contrast the chaotic image of a mind without a center, proposed by the neurosciences, with the event of unity in diversity, compatible with the philosophical position that it is possible to naturalize consciousness and, at the same time, recognize it as a cornerstone of our conceptions of the world, namely, the expression of a single and continuous subject over time. In this systemic vision, therefore, the concept of plasticity confers uniqueness and irreducibility upon the subject who thinks in a continuous circularity between what is given (genetic level) and what is in continuous becoming (epigenetic level). Thus, maintaining neo-connectionism and the contemporary theory of complexity in its classic version as a theoretical point of reference, Siegel considers the brain as a dynamic system formed of neural networks that can be activated in an infinite number of patterns and of different "neural profiles" and that they can remember and learn from past experiences making the probability of certain patterns of excitation increase (Siegel, 1995, 1996). It is what Siegel defines as "experience dependent cerebral development," that is to say a development which strongly characterizes the first years of life and lasts throughout the arc of existence, influencing not only moments of memorization and learning but also recuperation and use of cognitive-relational skills. Therefore, in Siegel's opinion memory is an active set of processes. In fact, even the recalling of an architectural structure is actually a dynamic representational processes. Since remembering is not the reactivation of an old engram, but "*it is the construction of a new neural net profile with features of the old engram and elements of memory from other experiences, as well as influences from the present state of mind*" (Siegel 1999, p. 28). Also differentiated are the processes that make "sense" of human experience: these processes include an increase in excitability and neuronal activation, an increase in neuronal plasticity and the creation of new synaptic connections as well as the creation of new circuits that link different brain areas. Thus the neurobiological level is designed to deal with various energetic forces and modulate them in relation to different experiences. At their basis, these are organized into the three previously mentioned fields (memory, attachment and emotions), which , following in Siegel's steps, we are preparing to examine in more detail.

In the first place, the treatment of the functions of *memory* considers three aspects: the distinction between explicit and implicit memory, the capacity to produce associations between different kinds of experiences and the space-time integration dimension that our mind possesses. For this investigation the third aspect is particularly important and brings Siegel to underline the acquisition of autonoetic conscience as a fundamental moment in children's development.

Noetic consciousness (knowing the fact that one was once in a particular place) is different from autonoetic consciousness (recalling the self's experience of the trip), both in subjective experience and in the involvement of the prefrontal cortices in the latter process. In fact, episodic recall activates autobiographical memory representations and evokes a process of mental time travel (the sense of the self in time). The distinct experiential aspects of memory are thought to involve different centers of activation within the brain (for example, semantic recall appears to involve a dominance of left over right hippocampal activation, while autobiographical recall involves more of the right hippocampus and right orbitofrontal cortex). Though semantic and episodic memory have much in common—due to their flexible accessibility and their virtual unlimited capacities for representing data—they appear to be mediated by distinct mechanisms (Siegel, 2006). Regarding the function of episodic memory, there appears to be a much larger process involved than merely the autobiographical content of representations of personally experienced events. In other words, autonoetic awareness involves the experience of mental time travel and is directly linked to the processes of the prefrontal regions of the brain. While autonoetic consciousness is created within the various layers of prefrontal function, these include an integrating capacity (in which more recently stored information can be organized and sequenced into a meaningful set of representations), executive functions (which provide a more global control of widely distributed brain processes) and the mediation of self-reflection and social cognition (Siegel, 1999, 2001). Siegel's evolutionary description focuses on the gradual acquisition of the sense of self and others in time thanks to the formation and progressive refinement of space-time integration skills that the adult mind possesses. Skills that are expressed and nurtured for example in the processes of narration and self-narration, aimed exactly at creating temporal sequences that are coherent and convincing for those who think, create, listen or share. From this viewpoint then he explains that the brain responds to experience by establishing connections among neurons and that those pathways activated simultaneously become associated with one another and are more likely to be activated together again in the future. Before the development of the hippocampus (medial temporal lobe), the brain is only able to have implicit memory; this diverse form of memory is thought to include behavioral, emotional, perceptual, and possibly somatosensory memory and merely creates the mental experience of behavior, emotion, or perception (Siegel, 1999, 2001, 2007).

> During the second year of life, the hippocampus matures enough for a second form of memory to become available. Explicit memory requires focal attention for encoding and leads to the long-term and then permanent accessibility of elements of first factual and later autobiographical memory. The encoding of explicit memory, which is dependent upon the hippocampus, yields a form of retrieval that involves the sense of recollection—and, if autobiographical, of the self at some time in the past. [. . .] The autobiographical narrative process is directly influenced by both implicit and explicit memory. [. . .]As the child develops into the third year of life, the orbitofrontal cortex becomes capable of mediating episodic memory or autonoesis. In a fundamental manner, the narrative process allows individuals to shape the flow of information about the self and others" (Siegel, 1999, pp. 64–66).

Moreover, we have the phenomena of attachments that are the first place to experience the tight interconnection between the physical and psychical forces of a relationship. If attachment is based on a relationship of reciprocity transmitted via language during the first phases of development, parent and child enter in a kind of emotional synergy where it is possible to perceive the intended meanings of the other. The ability of the parent to elaborate the messages transmitted by the child and to respond in an adequate manner are fundamental conditions for the establishment of collaborative communication within the couple that is the basis of safe attachment (Bowlby, 1988, 1979; Santerini, 2011). In relation to this, Siegel states that the need for this type of communication and connection may not end with childhood (Siegel, 1999, 2001). Hence, the possibility of thinking of synaptic plasticity and neural development as shaped by the branches of affective relationships. Emotional attachments are, in fact, real relational processes between the person and the environment, processes, i.e., able to qualify the intentionality and clarify the values and even to illuminate rationality itself. Thus, the educational fields and, in particular, the classroom must be included as places where the cognitive dimension (*logos*) and affective (*eros*) are closely connected, effecting the integration "heart-hand-mind." According to Ainsworth (1978), the operational model of attachment is also translated into states of mind and objectively observable styles of relations. In light of all of this, therefore, Siegel (1999) speaks about "attunement" (a particular type of communication based on the facial expression, vocalizations, eye contact, and body gestures), which reveals the alignment of states of mind.

Further, we know that memory and the processes of attachment are associated with emotions understood, in agreement with Le Doux (1996) and Siegel (1995, 1996), as processes that involve the entire brain. So, we can think of emotions as dynamic phenomena created within cerebral processes of evaluation of meanings that are directly affected by social influences (Siegel, 2003). Emotions are studied by Siegel (1995, 2003) as energy flows or states of arousal and of activation that involve the brain and other systems of the organism and, at the level of the mind, influence the processing of information through the processes of selection of meaning. Siegel's observations about potential emotional exchanges have a deep importance. The primary emotions are associated with states of mind that change in time according to an informational flow that is unique each time (as only one of its kind is the way in which they are expressed in each moment). The selection of stimuli and the relative attribution of meaning are the primary functions of emotional processes. Various studies have identified the orbitofrontal area of the cerebral cortex as being involved in processes of evaluation-selection, processing the semantics of sensorial perception, emotional modulation and attention holding. Moreover, the orbitofrontal area of the cerebral cortex is between "lower" regions (involved in receiving input from the body and the senses) and the "higher" parts, involved in integrating information and creating elaborate thoughts. It must be considered that the orbitofrontal cortex is responsible for a progress consisting of taking changing or unexpected internal and external conditions and responding through new and flexible behavior (this progress is called "response flexibility"). Therefore, the prefrontal cortex plays a crucial role in attention and the emotions, allowing responses that reflect the significance of sensory events and not their superficial characteristics; moreover, the prefrontal mediation of response flexibility enables new and personally meaningful responses to be enacted (Siegel, 1999). Response flexibility and narrative coherence reveal important comparisons with the functions of the prefrontal cortex in relation to attachment modes, experience dependent ways of developing, and modes of personal interaction. On the relationship between emotions and cerebral asymmetry many theories have been proposed (Siegel, 1999; Damasio, 1999; Edelman, 2006; Freeman, 2004). Even though many now agree that the processes of evaluation and arousal involve the entire brain, subjective experience and the nature of the emotions in the two hemispheres can be quite different (Freeman, 2009; Siegel, 2007). It would be reasonable to propose that subjective awareness and the expression of what we have defined as primary emotions are mediated by the non-verbal right hemisphere, even though it is probable that both hemispheres participate in producing these emotions. According to Freeman and Siegel, the same processes create emotion and meaning. Information processing involves the creation and manipulation of cognitive representations, while the latter directs the flow of information processing.

> Within perception and memory, the appraisal systems of the brain must label representations as significant or value-laden. In this way, the appraisal and arousal processes—the central features of emotion—are interwoven with the representational processes of 'thinking.' *Creating artificial or didactic boundaries between thought and emotion obscures the experiential and neurobiological reality of their inseparable nature*" (Siegel, 1999, p. 159).

The neuroscientific revaluation of the emotions offered by Siegel, therefore, sheds new light on the issue concerning the nature and development of the human mind, pushing towards a non-reductionist naturalistic solution whereby the origin of subjective consciousness (and therefore also of the moral sense) would lie in the emotional conditions in which human life is born and in which only it is possible (Di Francesco, 1998; Salmeri, 2013). Such conditions would translate into ethical attitudes when they are mediated by symbolic language and thought, namely, by the emergence of a narrative identity as a meeting point between the descriptive and prescriptive, between what you can and what you must, between action and ethics. The story is exactly what weaves and leads to unity the fragments of life, emotion and experience that accumulate, in search of the meaning of our existence (Santerini, 2011). We are now in front of the main topic of the present volume: the capacity of regulating the emotions in relation to the formation of the self. While referring to Siegel's considerations, we are going to continue this interdisciplinary path trying to investigate the mystery of the sense of self through the languages and methodologies of different disciplines such as psychology, the educational sciences, neurobiology and cognitive neuroscience, arriving, at the end, to highlight the epistemological implications of this systemic and non-standard approach. Taking inspiration from models of the mind that are fundamentally based on the systemic metaphor, Siegel considers the mind as a complex structure able to represent and process information, to sustain composite processes of co-operative communication—the co-construction of meanings—and dynamics of conscious thinking and affection:

> the mind constructs its own experience of reality. Emanating from the interface of the brain and human relationships, the mind creates connections among the various elements of representations, ranging from sensations and images to concepts and words. The connections among the layers of neural activity weave a fabric of subjective life: They enable us to feel, behave, think, plan, and communicate" (Siegel, 1999, pp. 204–205).

Then, the capacity to reflect on the placement of the self along an axis of integration and temporal development should be considered a highly evolved form of consciousness. In function of exactly this level of the mind, the qualitative ways of accessing information and the subjective qualities of experience are seen, by some scholars, as the two dimensions that are typical of *conscience*. The formulation and management of emotions and the attribution of meaning to these latter instead involves both hemispheres, even though the qualitative ways in which each hemisphere is influenced by these neuronal activations is different (Damasio, 2007, 2010).

As we have shown in the last paragraph of the previous chapter, both the cognitive sciences and the studies of child development seem to suggest the existence in each of us of various selves (or states of self) characterized by internal cohesion and continuity in time (Damasio, 2010; Zeki, 2011; Siegel, 2001, 2003). Through the regulation of internal and external factors the system of the mind evolves with the emergence of a series of states of self which possess their own cohesion and continuity. Mind, as a non-linear system, is able to vary these constraints rapidly, with a distinct and discontinuous activation of the states of self: the creation of a stable and coherent complex from the different states of self is one of the central objectives of emotional development and the processes of self-regulation (Siegel, 2006). In each moment a state of mind emerges from the infinitary spectrum of "adjacent possible" brain activities that groups a coherent ensemble of processes directed at reaching specific objectives and the integration of these processes is mediated by the emotions (Kauffman, 2005). So, emotions constitute, according to Ciompi (1991) and Siegel (1995), "organizational and integrative processes" that a) confer specific meanings and motivational direction on stimuli; b) connect mental processes that are synchronically and diachronically distinct, creating complex associations between abstract representational processes that present significant emotional analogues; and c) participate in state-dependent processes of memory, synchronizing, on the basis of past experiences, the activity of the whole organism in function of the particular needs of the moment.

Thus, in agreement with Siegel's research (2006), we can infer that the modulation of processes of evaluation-selection and arousal plays a key role in the organization of the mind. Collaborative forms of communication and "reflexive dialogues," which emerge in secure attachment relationships, give the ability to the child to regulate the emotions, allowing him or her to develop internal coherence and mentalized functions (Siegel, 2003). Siegel considers auto-regulation and the regulation of the emotions to be practically synonymous because he retains that emotions are integrative processes that connect all the functions and activities of the mind. Emotions can be defined as subjective experiences that involve neurobiological, experiential and behavioral components and therefore the level of emotional communication is of fundamental importance. Through this the minds of two individuals can enter into connection, establishing attachment phenomena essential for the growth of brain structures oriented to reciprocal self-regulation (Siegel, 2001). Siegel (1999, 2007) considers the integration of the mind as directly connected to the integration of the various co-existent selves and the integration of the various states of self brings psychological wellbeing but at the same time new adaptive capacities distinct from the various selves; thus, synchronic integration involves elements that create a cohesive mental state. Various aspects of neural activity are clustered together within a functional state of mind as a part of vertical, dorsal–ventral, and lateral integration in a given moment. Therefore, Siegel suggests that at another level, as the individual's states of mind flow across time, diachronic integration "links" these together in a manner that facilitates flexible and adaptive functioning (spatio-temporal integration). This type of integration serves as a mechanism of self-regulation, it serves to organize the flow of states (Siegel, 1999). In the quality of autobiographical narrations we can observe the level of coherence reached by the mind and the flexibility of the adaptive capacities of the various selves as well as their coefficient of stability. The quality of these cognitive processes can be analyzed both in terms of synchronous integration, complexity—understood as the existence of various symbolic-semantic levels—and diachronic integration—understood as the duration, articulation and coherence of the temporal sequence (Sbattella 2006; Santerini, 2011).

The integration of the self is a complex dynamic which creates coherence through deep processes of self-organization linked to interactions with other selves (Zeki, 1999; Freeman, 2000b). This is a nonlinear process that goes through regressive and progressive moments; it is the result of organizational, disorganizational and reorganizational processes (Atlan, 1998). According to Siegel (2007) the integration processes allow the establishment of a sense of congruence and unity within flexible patterns in the flow of energy and information: this is the consistency of the mind. Differently, dissociation is defined clinically in terms of the compromising of the integrative mechanisms that involve the various mental processes such as, for example, perception, memory, identity and conscience. In some cases the conflict between needs and different states of the self can bring about internal or external difficulties that generate a dysfunctional picture, which is why the mind needs to master adaptive capacities (Sbattella, 2006). Siegel concludes his book highlighting, once again, the role of integration processes and their relation with the processing of resonance emphasizing the nature of optimal experiences for the growth of the capacity of auto-regulation and integration. In Siegel's opinion if "integration" is the process that creates coherence in the mind, "coherence" is the state of the system in which many layers of neural functioning become activated and "cohere" to each other over time. He further suggests that the complexity theory gives an insight into the reason why this linking process may occur: by maximizing complexity, the states of the system achieve stability. Thus, the mind recruits various layers of processes into a cohesive state of mind (namely, a state in which subcomponents become linked together at a given moment), moving to complexity, therefore, as the mind emerges across time, cohesive states become a part of a coherent flow. The process of integration

> recruits differentiated subcomponent circuits into a larger functional system through a fundamental reentry process. The co-regulating, mutually influencing state of reentrant connections is called 'resonance.' In other words, *integration utilizes the resonance of different subsystems to achieve cohesive states and a coherent flow of states across time. Such a process creates a more complex, functionally linked system, which itself can become a subcomponent of even larger and more complex systems*" (Siegel, 1999, pp. 321–322).

It is in "peak experiences," experiences characterized by a sense of "union" that the individual feels a part of a process that goes beyond the limits of the self. Such experiences offer an empirical support to the idea of the existence of a relationship between experiences of union-flow and integrative processes. Narrative experience occupies a significant position amongst these peak experiences with regards to integration of the self. The recall mechanisms of the autobiographical memory are all processes mediated principally by the right hemisphere. This hemisphere is further majorly implicated in the representational capacity of states of mind and it is therefore probable that it carries out a dominant role in self-reflexive functions proper to the processes of interiorization (Siegel, 1995, 1996).

According to Sbattella (2006) and Santerini (2011) narrative processes involve different ways to process information: perceptive representations, analogue, context dependent, autonoetics and right hemisphere mentalizing contribute in large measure to the themes and imaginary content of narrative processes; the logical and linear interpretation of these representations and the communication of these narrative details is based instead on the deductive and linguistic capacities and the representations of the left hemisphere. So, remembering and narrating contribute to a new structuring of events which exploits new contexts and conscious and unconscious components (Siegel, 2001). Bilateral integration mechanisms can be the basis of various creative processes. The acquisition of a greater capacity of interpersonal connection transforms one's "state of mind with respect to attachment." According to Siegel (1999, 2001), the capacity to experience and appreciate more articulate and intense sensations and emotions gives new vitality and creativity in relation to the development of integration mechanisms which allow greater resonance between the various information processing methods. Many of these processes remain unconscious (non-declarative memory) but can give rise to the awareness of a new flow of coherent activations within the mind (self-organization and re-organization processes):

> Such vibrant connections between minds can be seen within various kinds of emotional relationships, such as those of romantic partners, friends, colleagues, teachers and students, therapists and patients, and parents and children. Two people become companions on a mutually created journey through

> time. Interpersonal integration can be seen in spontaneous, resonant communication that flows freely and is balanced between continuity, familiarity, and predictability on one side and flexibility, novelty, and uncertainty on the other. [. . .] When such a process is in full activation, the vital feeling of connection is exhilarating. When interpersonal communication is 'fully engaged'—when the joining of minds is in full force—there is an overwhelming sense of immediacy, clarity, and authenticity. It is in these heightened moments of engagement, these dyadic states of resonance, that one can appreciate the power of relationships to nurture and to heal the mind" (Siegel, 1999, pp. 335–337).

From this perspective, therefore, it is possible to understand more deeply the decisive role played by education (epigenetic level)—powered by the emotional aspects and guided by the awareness of how humans recognize themselves as such also through functions such as mirror neurons, functions, namely, interpretable as neurological references of empathy—at the level of building the structures of knowledge and the formation of sense of self. Hence the need, through the educational process, to reinforce the original compassion based on the innate capacity of imitation with behaviors of aid and cooperation, "orienting ourselves to be not only naturally, but also culturally, *in* others and *for* others" (Santerini, 2011, p. 208).

4.2 Mirror neurons and empathy

This book, through neurobiological and theoretical-epistemological reflections on some of the recent discoveries in the neurosciences has shown up to this point how much it is realistically and scientifically possible to definitively overcome the traditional mind/body dichotomy and causal concepts based on a before and an after, such as "psycho-somatic" or "somato-psychic" (Freeman, 2000a; Siegel, 1999, 2007). The resolute emancipation from this dividing of the living world into discrete units, indeed, has often risked stopping at the formulation of a noble intention or utopian visions. That is why, from my point of view, facing this need in the first place signifies having the epistemological awareness that it is no longer possible to adopt the categories of "mind" and "body" in the traditional and ontological sense. A study of the mind/body question which does not include a concept of relation is revealed to be naive and scientifically inadequate (Giannone, Lo Verso, 1996; Siegel, 1999). Results from the field of complexity theory have, as we have seen, rendered materialistic monism and individualistic reductionism obsolete, but recently they have also touched on the field of cognitive neuroscience, by virtue of its attempt to connect neuronal development with the web of human relational experiences through which we gradually realize ourselves. Siegel (2001, 2006), as we have said above, writes that the mind is a product of interactions between interpersonal experience and the structure and function of the brain, but his relational position hardens when he sustains that human connections mold the nervous connections which give origin to the mind. Therefore important results at the psychiatric level, contributions from complexity theory and the constructivist model (when it looks at psychodynamic valence), as well as the evolution of the neurosciences and cognitive psychology have contributed to the creation of a mind-body model which neither amalgamates nor separates the three aspects of the mind-body-relation problem, but instead sees them as three points of observation, each of which can and sometimes must be privileged at different times. (Freeman, 1994, 2004, 2007; Siegel, 1995; Edelman, Tononi, 2000; Edelman, 2004, 2006). This is a paradigm that until a short time ago did not appear capable of holding the various aspects of the question together but now seems sufficiently powerful and complex enough both in theoretical and epistemological terms to be a useful basis for further research.

The greater agreement between neo-connectionist (and post-cognitivist) epistemology and neurobiology have started a paradigm shift that has assumed the shape of an interdisciplinary hybrid, fundamental for the understanding of the nexuses between relational and corporeal processes. Taking care not to uncritically overlay concepts we can nevertheless say that on the basis, above all of Kandel and Squire's research (2009), the conceptualization around the "Self" currently also includes molecular biology and immunology (Ammaniti, 1989; Fasolo *et al.*, 2005; Rispoli, Andriello, 1988). In confirmation of this, the most recent research in neurobiology (Owen et al., 2005; Owen et al., 2009), using a multidisciplinary approach that has contributions from psychology, psychiatry and philosophy of the mind (Searle, 2004, 2008; Nagel, 1978, 2012), has tried to develop the theme of original intersubjectivity of the human mind from a cerebral point of view, that is to say what the subjective group analysis calls "transpersonal." This is understood by Lo Verso (1989, 1994) as the ensemble of relations within a specific cultural system that the individual incorporates dynamically from birth onwards; and therefore includes constituent information on the anthropological-psychic side, psychic birth and therefore the personality. An ever greater part of the neurosciences holds that the brain is a plastic organ, open to experience, capable, therefore of assuming different structural and functional connotations according to the genetic and experiential bases that characterize a single person. This plastic conception (and in some senses also dynamic-experiential) of the brain is of central importance to us because as we will see next, it creates possible alignments and compatibility with the results of research in the bioeducational sciences. This orientation, as known to the scientific world and beyond goes by the name of *Neural Darwinism* (Edelman, 1987, 1990, 2004).

Edelman's by-now classic theory of the mental is based on the assertion that the brain develops by creating connections between neurons from the embryo onwards: from the potentially practically infinite network of neural connections each individual develops some but not others (the phenomena of neuronal pruning), in response to sensorial stimuli. The neural makeup is therefore influenced from the first months of life by the external world. The partial cultural influence with respect to genes allows each of us a subjective moment of development at the brain level too. In substance this new paradigm finally allows a more precise hypothesis of how neuronal plasticity and culture can weave together to create intelligence. On this subject the studies of brain structure and function continuously supply new and more accurate indications of the mechanisms through which experiences influence man's mental processes (Kandel, 2005; Milner, Squire, Kandel 1998). Substantially the mind should not be understood in terms of structure, but rather as a dynamic process that emerges from the activity of the brain whose structure and functions are directly influenced by interpersonal experiences (Siegel, 1999). In particular the mind develops from processes that regulate energy flows and information within the brain and between different brains (Siegel, 1999; Freeman, Vitiello, 2008; Carsetti, 2009a). The concept of the mind as an entity therefore needs revision. The mind is not a thing or object located in the body or space but a line used to circumscribe numerous psychological processes, mental phenomena and different personal experiences, even if they are often connected. The time in which we could talk about the mind or the brain and their causal interactions is past; today we occupy ourselves with a variety of mental–cerebral phenomena and their relationships. The multiplicity of mental processes is usually indicated as the mind and functions at a higher level of biological organization than the brain. A lot of scientific literature indicates that the development of the brain is the product of the effects that experiences have on the expression of genetic potential (Benedersky, Lewis, 1994; Goldsmith et al., 1997). Human DNA is formed by genes which in turn contain the information that allows cellular neurons to differentiate, develop and die, during the construction of brain circuits. For Siegel (1996) these are processes that, while genetically programmed, are at the same time "experience dependent."

Genes carry out two key functions for the development of human life (Kandel, 1998). The first refers to their ability to allow the transmission of genetic information from one generation to the next. The second function which operates at an ontogenetic level refers to their capacity to determine the type of protein synthesized in a cellular setting. This second function can be notably influenced by the experience each human has in the world: human experiences are able to directly influence the transcription and therefore the ways in which genes are expressed through protein synthesis (Siegel, 1999). As for the brain, this means that experiences can have direct effects on the processes that bring about the development of neuronal circuitry, inducing the formation of new synaptic connections, modifying the pre-existing ones and favoring their elimination (Kandel, 1989, 1998; Post, Weiss, 1997). In the course of the neural development of the child, the social world represents the principal source of experiences that influence genetic expression. Changes induced at the level of genetic transcription provoke structural modifications of nerve cells, thus molding the "relational mind." In turn, the activity of the mind brings about physiological variations in the brain that can lead to the expression of different genes (Siegel, 1999, 2003). The mind in all of its stages of life and phases of development can modify the structures, functions and neuro-anatomical connections of the brain. This constant plasticity is connected in various ways to the mind's *radically relational essence* which continually constructs structural pairings with the environmental system (Napolitani, 1987), that is to say new combinations between things in the world which give rise to an incessant psychic dynamism. The link, at the neuronal level, of man's relational essence as indicated by a large clinical-epistemological literature is represented by mirror neurons (Rizzolatti, Fogassi, Gallese, 2002, 2006), particular kinds of neurons that are *activated* both when a person carries out a certain action and when he observes it being carried out by others. It will be fundamentally important for post-cognitivist psychology to have data that tells us what happens in terms of mirror neurons when *mirroring* takes place in the mind of the person who thinks, imagines, desires and daydreams a relational moment with another person (Foulkes, 1975), as well as when this happens in a dream. The question arises because notoriously the imagination creates identification with things imagined. On the level of actions, furthermore, these neurons make it possible to immediately gather the emotional reactions of others. In substance, the discovery of mirror neurons has brought to light how the reciprocity that ties us to others is a natural, prelinguistic, pre-conceptual and pre-rational human condition (Rizzolatti, Sinigaglia, 2006, 2008). This seems to suggest that they represent a necessary but not sufficient prerequisite for empathetic behavior between people, and vice versa that this is linked, in its reality to experiences. Sharing at a visceral-motor level in the emotional state of another is different from being empathetic to them (Rizzolatti, Sinigaglia, 2007, 2010). For the "system mechanism" mirror neurons do not always correspond to empathy for the other; rather, this possibility and more generally the numerous ways of feeling the other also and above all have to do with the relational quality that links people, from my point of view, with their identity understood subjectively. Conversely, for two people to establish a full and efficient emotional communication, it is necessary for each of them to allow their state of mind to be influenced by the other, thus "feeling" them and getting on their wavelength. The axiom that is the basis of this book springs from this, that the "relation" (or rather the "intentionality," as Freeman would have it) is the basis of the living world (and therefore of every educational project). It is clear that the relationship between mirror neurons and psycho-relational facts still needs to be better understood as regards various aspects, for example, the symbolic, the emotions, mental reprocessing, meanings attributed to others' emotions and the role of the familiar and culture in forming the mirror neuron system. This last point is particularly important. According to Iacoboni (2008), the activity of mirror neurons[1] recalls primary intersubjectivity (Trevarthen, 1996), that is to say the first capacity of interaction that the child reveals and develops in interactions with its "caregivers." Essentially mirror neurons form and grow during and thanks to these first key relationships and, from our point of view, the discourse can be widened to all the significant relationships (internal and external) that man experiences daily. In this sense Iacoboni writes:

> Although it is likely that some mirror neurons are functioning very early in life and facilitate the earliest interactions, I believe that most of our mirror neuron system is actually formed during the months and years of such interactions. The shaping of mirror neurons in the baby's brain is especially likely to happen during reciprocal imitation [. . .]. If mirror neurons are actually shaped in our brain by the coordinated activities of mother and father and baby, then these cells not only embody both self and the other, but start doing so at a time when the baby has more of an undifferentiated sense of us than any sense of an independent self, before the baby can pass the mirror recognition test. From this primary 'us,' however, the baby slowly but surely comes to perceive the other naturally and directly, and obviously without any complex inference; it proceeds to carve out a proper sense of self and other. How? With the help of a special type of mirror neurons, which I called super mirror neurons. (Iacoboni, 2008, pp. 155–156).

Well, he continues, super mirror neurons seem to be cells that

> have a very interesting pattern of neuronal firing. The firing rate increases while the patient performs the action, as in monkeys. In sharp contrast with mirror neurons in monkeys, however, these cells shut down entirely while the patient observes the action. This pattern of activity suggests that these cells may have an inhibitory role during action observation. By shutting themselves down, they may tell the more classical mirror neurons that the observed action should not be imitated. Furthermore, this differential coding for action of the self (increased firing rate) and for actions of others (decreased firing rate) may represent a wonderfully simple neural distinction between self and other implemented by these special types of super mirror neurons. [. . .]Indeed, the brain areas from which we recorded these cells are the least developed in early infancy and show the most dramatic developmental changes later on (pp. 202–203).

What Iacoboni sustains is very significant for us, above all for its connection with the organismic vision of the bio-educative sciences that I will soon present. Nevertheless for now it seems clear to us that the system of mirror neurons seems to represent in large part the neurobiological connection with the assumptions of the theory of intentionality as proposed by Freeman, a theory that has shone a light deep into the relational essence of the human identity. Obviously this discourse is not exclusive to the complexity paradigm. Focusing attention on the field of psychotherapy, indeed, the relationship between mirror neurons and psycho–relational facts, and therefore neuro-relational processes that these intertwinings imply on the symbolic and emotional plane assumes central importance. It is most significant in this sense that mirror neurons and perhaps all brain activity in general are activated both by external events and imagined ones (Oliverio, 2008, 2013). This clarifies a question that we previously asked ourselves. Thought, fantasy and even dreams when ("quite often") concentrated on external experiences (and therefore on relations with others), probably activate neuronal events even in the absence of a real interpersonal experience, that is to say that maybe activation could be connected to an interiorized or fantasized relationship. From this point of view the inquiry into the destination of emotional-relational experiences that are lived unconsciously is fascinating. We are not talking about a question stimulated by a whim since great importance has been given to unconscious (or unaware) processes by all the fields that take inspiration from the neurosciences or psychological research (Oliverio, Ferraris, 2007; Kandel, 2005). Reflections on interiorized unconscious relations are in line with what the mirror neuron system reveals. Their discovery testifies indeed to how rooted, deep and indispensable the link with another is to a human being and how bizarre it is to conceive of an I without a you, or without an us (Rizzolatti, 2005; Sinigaglia, Rizzolatti, 2011); this goes for comprehension of human nature as well as the epistemological-theoretical decisions for curing psychic disturbance (Lo Coco, Lo Verso, 2006). There is then a "quality" of our inner life, a phenomenal dimension that manifests itself externally and that the eye of the observer in a more or less accurate manner can read and understand. Over the course of the history of human thought there have been various attempts to identify this transfer of significance that is pre-predicative, pre-verbal and implicit. One way to understand this could be, for example the following passage from *Aurora* by Nietzsche:

> To understand the other, that is to imitate their sentiments in ourselves, we place ourselves in a viewpoint of internal imitation that somehow gives rise to, leads to a gushing of analogous sentiments in us, by virtue of an ancient association between movement and sensation" (Nietzsche, 1881).

Mirror neurons, from a certain point of view exemplify this relationship between movement and sensation.

Another fundamental contribution is that of phenomenology. Husserl is a complex author that has been criticized for transcendental solipsism, underlining Cartesian aspects. Above all in the conclusive phase of his thought the need to understand the intersubjective dimension, underlining its centrality in the definition of conscious subjectivity emerges ever more evidently. Particularly interesting is the Husserlian concept of "paarung" according to which the Other is understood thanks to a primitive holistic process of coupling. In my opinion it seems like a good point of departure to point to the implicit dimension of the intersubjective capacity to transfer meanings from one person to another using the body as a vehicle of this transfer, both from the point of view of expression of significance and the capacity to decode it when we are spectators. In phenomenology the crucial dimension of intersubjectivity in the construction of subjectivity is underlined; which does not mean that subjectivity does not have its own pregnant, founding and extremely important dimension. They are two complementary dimensions but if we leave intersubjectivity out we risk falling back on the image of the mind and the psycheism that has prevailed and characterized the cognitive sciences over the last fifty years, that is to say that reifies the body. A body which is the pre-logical and pre-predicative origin of our capacity for comprehension, "flesh of the world" as Merleau-Ponty writes (1942, 1945, 1964), underlining the centrality of empathy in experiencing the world. *Einfuhlung*, empathy is also seen by Sigmund Freud as a fundamental mechanism for transferring inter-individual significance. In 1921 the father of psychoanalysis wrote: "One path leads from identification, through imitation to empathy, that is to say the understanding of the non-propositionality of social cognition." (Gallese, 2007, pp. 2–3). In the face of the phenomenon of empathy these authors do not refer to a series of behaviors or functions but to experience, to what Edith Stein meant when she talked about the "making present of the other's experience," that grasping of the others' humanity through an intentional act which goes beyond observation or cognition, recalling us to Stein's works (1917). Thompson considers empathy as "a unique and irreducible form of intentional experience":

> although it is based on a sensitive perception and can include inference (in difficult or problematic situations), this is never reducible to the sum of the two planes [. . .]. Rather we have experience of the other as a whole through empathy [. . .]. When we see another person we do not perceive their body only as a physical thing but as a living body equal to ours. Empathy is not simply grasping the specific experiences of

> another person (sadness, joy and so on) but is experiencing the other as a whole" (Thompson, 2001, p. 16).

Even Varela in the neurobiological study of empathy does not see it as a feeling or a particular kind of understanding, but as our fundamental way of "being with others," of "the fact of being structurally conceived to have relationships with our kin, individuals of the same species."

> One of the most important discoveries of the phenomenological movement is that the investigation of the structure of human experience leads inevitably to a change of viewpoints in the consideration of the unbreakable ties that bind us in an empathetic mesh, my conscience of others and of the world of phenomena" (Varela, Shear, 1999, p. 46). Just as for Husserl recognition of the other passes through the ambiguity of the body, Varela sees "embodiment" as the attempt to "render intelligible the fact that an entity can have both material and mental characteristics despite the apparent difference between the two" (Varela, Shear, 1999).

In a similar[2] way to Husserl he finds in this "lived duality" the source of recognition of the other: if the body is an "ontological machine," an ambiguous unity of mechanism and transcendence, "one must abandon the notion of internal as a logical system and external as a source of information" and admit the co-existence of many *possible worlds.* Here Varela specifies, "We are not talking about philosophy but a logic of research" (Varela, 1990, p. 46).

Finally, Gallese, in presenting the results on mirror neurons (1996, 2008, 2009), affirms that his notion of "incarnate simulation" is linked to "how we are made" (Gallese, 2006, p. 315). This direction of research is motivated by an idea whose origins lie in the founder of phenomenology: to promote a science of the world of life, a science of experience; that which follows therefore is not just a formal functioning of the theories but getting close to the truth of what we are. That is why as Gallese says "important aspects of phenomenological reflection have found confirmation in the results of neuroscientific research of intersubjectivity" (p. 293). These are reciprocal confirmations from different viewpoints that aim to know the "lived experience of reality." Exactly this exploratory behavior of empathy shows it is reasonable that "the coming together of neuroscience and phenomenology can help us to better understand essential aspects of intersubjectivity" (p. 294).

Contrary to the cognitivist theory of the mind which holds understanding of the other as dependent on inferential and logical processes, the discovery of mirror neurons supports the hypothesis that when we have dealings with others we recognize them as being similar to ourselves and we can understand them before any interpretation. This process indeed, in line with the phenomenological analysis is "embodied and pre-declarative" (p. 316). Again: the phenomenological digging carried out by Stein on empathy encounters its limits as is made clear by Ales Bello:

> When I enter into contact with that which I consider separate to me but similar to me, alter ego, I understand, intuit, comprehend and therefore empathize with what they are living; in this comprehension I realize that he is living for example an emotion, but he is living it himself or herself as a completely original fact, but not original for me; I empathize with his situation but certainly do not live the contents of his experience which is incommunicable" (Ales Bello, 1999, p. 72–73).

In line with the phenomenological analysis Gallese's research shows that different cortical circuits are activated when I act compared with those that are activated when another carries out the same action and the activation is of different intensity. The "system of shared multiplicity" described by the Italian academic indeed, "doesn't imply that we experience others as we experience ourselves. This system simply constitutes and promotes the process of mutual intelligibility" (Gallese, 2006, p. 318). "Simply" the scientific studies that are inspired by the phenomenological method confirm that, if we remain faithful to who we are, empathy is not any old psychological phenomena to be explained within various theoretical frameworks, but the very possibility of intersubjective communication.

In the light of all this I allow myself to close this paragraph with the following consideration of Armezzani:

Not only ethical behavior but also science is based on recognition of the other: all of knowledge is based on meeting the presence of the other, on that original otherness that marks our life from its first stages. What Maturana (1975, 1978) called 'structural coupling' and Husserl (1931), with an analogous term called *Paarung*, expresses that original and continuous interaction with the world of experience in which we immediately meet the other as 'validator'; from the first relationships of the new born with the mother to formal scientific communications the other is the testing ground of our ideas about the world. That is why it's necessary to definitively abandon the behavior of the disinterested observer from a distance of 'these strange objects of study' and to start considering ourselves as belonging to the same tribe, like someone who speaks the same language and shares the same codes" (Armezzani, 2008, p. 88).

4.3 Pedagogy between bio-neural sciences and philosophy

The change of paradigm in the field of neuroscience, the new frontiers opened by recent discoveries not only at a physiological level, but especially at an epigenetic level, have inspired, in pedagogy, new explorative dimensions in virtue of a gradual crossbreeding with biology and, in particular, with neuroscience; this latter process has favored the birth of a new interdisciplinary field of study. The bioeducational sciences (Frauenfelder, Santoianni, 2002, 2003b; Santoianni, Striano, 2003), understood as "a possible field of study containing within it pedagogy, neurosciences and post-cognitivism," aim for the realization of a synergetic vision able to ensure "non-reductive pedagogical approaches" and to interpret man in his intrinsic complexity. This is a new field of research containing within it various elements (epigenetic, biodynamic and synergetic) amongst which one, biodynamics, is preferentially oriented towards the problematic interaction between mind and body, between physical states and mental processes and between the structural and cognitive dimension of the subject. The biodynamic perspective therefore, recently redefined (Santoianni, Striano, 2003) more completely as one of the foundations of bioeducational sciences also includes within it a reference to an organismic concept ("organismic perspectives") of the subject (Frauenfelder, Santoianni, 1997; Frauenfelder et al., 2004; Damasio, 1994, 1999, 2010) through which the mind-body relation becomes a circular mind-brain-organism relationship. That is to say, the biological constitution of the individual, neural phenomena and neuro-regulatory circuits are constantly considered and explored without overlooking the reference to the organism in its complexity and systemic irreducible wholeness (Santoianni, 1998; Frauenfelder, 2001). It is from this perspective that the human brain and the rest of the body are considered to constitute a unique and inseparable organism united by biochemical processes. The complex and whole organism develops as an ensemble and interrelates constantly with the environment through forms of interaction that are not realized either just by the body or the mind: it is indeed the organism in its totality that encounters contextual variability (Edelman, 2006; Damasio, 1994, 2010). From this organismic perspective therefore

> the mind is *in the* body as well as being linked to the brain; but this body changes continuously, it transforms and develops following directions that can be different from individual to individual or can share characteristics. The mind is in the body but it is through the body that it can choose, interpret and produce complex orders of knowledge; the mind can develop theories, can recognize the implicit as well as the explicit character of thought, it can generate knowledge productively and independently, and yet it always does this on the basis of biologically rooted structures and functions. Structures and functions that justify thought even if the processes of consciousness do not necessarily arise from perceptive data of the mental representations, they are not predefinable and conserve adaptive characteristics (Fraunfelder et al., 2004, p. 60).

Through this viewpoint the structure function-synergy is expressed as a regulatory mechanism of the possible interactions between the organism and the environment (Frauenfelder, 1983, 1986, 2001). Both elements are in evolution continuously interacting with one another in a web of interdependence that is no longer possible to explain with the traditional nature/culture dichotomy (Jablonka, Lamb, 2005; Keller, 2000, 2010). Furthermore, conscience is no longer a computational product of the mind but the result of processes which imbues organismic corporeity and the representations that the brain activates regarding the organism in carrying out behaviors of actions; the mind, therefore, is linked to the brain but "lives" in a body (Sabatano, 2005). A body, in turn, occupies a space, lives in a time and moves in a place. Thus the studies of the mind *in vitro* become studies of the mind *in vivo,* and through this epistemological node one passes, gradually,

> from a computational, un-historic, decontextualised, rational and abstract image of the mind to the concept of *embodiment,* of corporeity and of the positioning of the mind *within* the body. Of 'incarnated' conscience; whence the concept of *embededdness,* of the rooting of the mind literally *within* the spatial and temporal situation. (Frauenfleder et al., 2004, p. 61).

All this has resulted in the identification of a sphere of research which, in passing from the pedagogy-biology relationship to that between pedagogy–neuroscience, marks out a new territory of research and is one of the major challenges today in the world of education.

> The challenge is to propose the definition of epistemological possibilities, interpretative co-ordinates and the operative methodologies of a scientific space in which educators, trainers, educationalists and researchers can collaborate. [. . .] It is ever more necessary therefore to identify research that can contribute to the bringing together of two worlds traditionally considered distant: pedagogy and the human sciences and the neurosciences and natural sciences, or as we would now say, sciences of the mind" (Frauenfelder et al., 2004, p. 6).

The plurality of meanings and levels through which research on learning potential and the functionality of the mind in the construction and management of knowledge can be classified around some thematic nuclei that could be seen as "universal joints" of training problems (pp. 6–7). These nuclei underline the interaction between the categories of quantity and quality, continuous and discontinuous, the stimulation of experience and the individual potential for learning. From this some general considerations emerge: each individual has a genetic potential to grow which is qualitatively and quantitatively different. Individual biological potential is not totally modifiable in epigenesis; the individual cognitive system manages to process input in a number of ways, which vary between individuals; as a result the function of an individual's cognitive system is in part general and in part specific, partly invariable and partly plastic (Kandel, 1976, 2005; Squire, Kandel, 2009). The function of the cognitive system is intimately linked to the affective-emotional dimension (Siegel, 1999) and even to the emotional and relational aspect of human life regulated by neuroanatomical structures and biochemical processes. Then, it is exactly through the analysis of the biological mechanism "that it is possible to give value to and enhance the incidence of the emotional element in the development of the human species" (Frauenfelder et al., 2004, p. 9).

The bioeducational sciences therefore constitute a multidisciplinary frontier which exercises a function of transfer and transversality in identifying a pedagogical direction common to various disciplines. These disciplines study the processes of evolutionary adaptation at the ontogenetic and phylogenetic levels, the integration and development of the adaptive system in the environment and the shared and situated dimension of knowing (Varela et al., 1991; Maturana, Varela, 1980, 1973) and other synergetic dynamics. The bioeducational sciences focus their research on identifying significant relationships between pedagogy, the biological sciences and the neurosciences in the paradigm of educational sciences and they express their meaning in the synergetic construction of the concept of *educability* towards the interpretative sphere of developmental pedagogy (Santoianni, 2006, 2012), with significant implications for the education sciences. In focusing on educability processes therefore a relationship between the individual, personal history, consolidation and transformation of experiences and synergetic interaction with the area of learning emerges (Sabatano 2004). Specifically, the memory and proto-memory are seen as multi-composite and multi-functional; modulated by various nuclei of activity, different between individuals both in a qualitative and evolutional senses, dynamic and subject to reshuffling and made up of and able to be separated from a number of points of view (cognitive, emotional, corporeal and perceptive). Therefore a consideration of memory that is of great interest to education emerges because one can hypothesize a relation between the ways that information is organized in an adaptive system and the ways this information is retrieved, the study of the ways through which information variables are conserved, processed and transformed could be a significant key to understand development processes of processing functions of adaptive systems and more generally, synergies that adaptive systems establish with the environments they interact with and together with which they are defined as organisms in development (Frauenfelder 1983). The multisystemic and constructive conception of the human memory describes memories as phenomena that are highly subjective to person and place; as a process therefore selective and individualistic put in play by the combined action of all the great cognitive functions: language, emotions, reasoning, the perceptive, sensorial and motor levels of the body and explicit and implicit knowledge. From this articulated and complex ensemble, multiple levels of memory and just as many mnestic sub-systems (implicit and explicit memory; semantic and episodic) arise, disseminated in various cerebral areas, plastically connected by synaptic circuitry and specific zones of convergence. Within this intricate ensemble of levels and systems the synchronic indicators of memory act (the affective sphere, the corporeal organismic level and the implicit dimensions of consciousness) that, combining with the various memories, modulate and organize the formation and the epigenetic development of the mnestic systems (Landry, Kandel, Rajasethupaty, 2013). Once the device that regulates the construction and evolution of the processes of memory is defined it is opportune, following Sabatano (2004), to concentrate our attention on the space of action that, within this process of formation is the role of education, that is to say, to establish what are the criteria of educability that can guide and promote educational practices.

The pedagogical necessities that seem to emerge in light of these considerations can help us create educational programs that recognize cognitive specificities and the systemic configurations of subjects; attentive to the sociocultural contexts in which they interact and to the relational and affective dynamics that operate in educational "settings"; sensitive to the most subtle and elusive nuances that are nevertheless strongly associated with educational practices (Frauenfelder, Santoianni, 2003b). One thinks, in that sense of implicit knowledge and proxemic levels of communication which act on the processes of construction of individual cognitive architecture. The construction of protomemory[3] training programs aims among other things to analyze the interaction between the memory and the specific emotional characteristics and cognitive configurations of various subjects in an evolutionary dimension. The way in which each individual uses his or her memory systems is influenced by individual cognitive and emotional factors, that is, vectors that are related to the analysis of characteristics that distinguish and differentiate the personal features of subjects in education, that constitute the backbone for the research into mnestic prerequisites of subjects as for example the sense of the real and the present, the use of experience, the control of the self, the metareflexive sense of responsibility, the capacity for cognitive and emotional decentering, initiative and the level of cognitive ability to change. According to Sabatano (2004, 2005), the analysis of these vectors constitutes the first factor of educability upon which it is possible to construct training programs to develop protomemory and create "body oriented mnestic programs," that is, spaces of learning in which the corporeal-organismic dimension is a lynchpin of the entire educational process, environments in which the body is considered as an open system in constant relation with an unspecified number of cooperating and interrelated agents (Sabatano, 2004). A "body oriented" training method therefore is interested in gathering what the body says about the mind, that is to say, in listening to the body in its way of presenting itself as an original phenomena, that is, before reading the contents it expresses. The third criteria of educability that regulates the putting together of a protocol record of the development of protomemory is related to the definition of preferential ways of mnestic coding that are enacted in children, ways that reflect the individual cognitive configurations, the combinations of the different types of intelligence in a particular individual which interface with mnestic coding channels that each subject preferentially employs and has available to process new information (Frauenfelder, 2001).

The definition of a multi-systemic conception of memory, supported by advances in neuroscience, seems to orient educational research to consider with growing interest the cognitive characteristics of the subject and the multiplicity of the factors in mnestic processes aimed at focusing on (antithetically to transmissive-imitative models of learning) the diversity of learning stimuli offered and the way in which, as a function of these the processing, modes of memory tend to vary (Santoianni, Sabatano, 2002). Whilst it is true that the management of learning communities should aim at giving value to the cognitive specificities and attitudes that each subject presents, it is also true that education as a global paedetic process can offer the subject in education continuous occasions for growth, sophistication and complexification of their thought processing modes, occasions also favored by the opportunity that the teacher can offer to accompany and implement the individual's preferential channels, with the acquisition, activation and appropriation of new and different channels of memorization (Sabatano, 2003). The construction of any educational project then cannot disregard the *eidos* of the human person (Agazzi, 1999; Armezzani et al., 2008).

This perspective invites us to rethink education and more generally the human sciences in virtue of an anthropological model which goes beyond the fragmentation of knowledge, a model that is capable of offering the scientific community cause for reflections difficult to classify in a single discipline. The questions regarding the essence of pedagogy and the educational sciences indeed immediately force us to rethink the anthropological horizon in a philosophical perspective where responsibility becomes the authentic measure of man. There is no doubt that the contribution of philosophy to pedagogy concerns the general aims of education. Specifically, the philosophy of education deals with epistemological and axiological aspects of education. The term "education" is polysemous and can indicate a philosophical system, an institution, a product, a political act or a system of management amongst other things. What does it mean to educate? The term "education" has a dual etymology: from the Latin *educere* (bring out) and *educare* (teach, raise, instruct). Furthermore, educating in the sense of development leads to taking care of the other. *Paideia,* the educational model of classical Athens, provided for the education of the young in two parallel branches: *therapeia,* which included the care of the body, and *epimeleia,* which included the care of the soul aimed to guarantee the harmonious socialization of the individual in the *polis* (Baccarini, 2003). Let us briefly consider both these aspects, reconnecting in part with what I have already examined. As regards the first, indeed, I refer to chapter one and the therapeutic effects of BCI (Brain Computer Interface), which represent an ample spectrum of solutions to acquire and process the commands originating from the brain through computerized instruments on patients in a vegetative or minimally conscious state. The most widely accepted definition of BCI was formulated by Wolpaw: "a direct brain-computer interface is a device that provides the brain with a new, non-muscular communication and control channel" (Cincotti et. al., 2007; Cincotti et al. 2008). Current systems mostly use electroencephalographs (EEG) that reveal the electric signal present on the scalp of the user and extract various physiological signals such as the evoked potential P300 or the voluntary activation related to "mental imagery." Through a phase of classification in "real time," these signals are recognized, discriminated and associated with commands to control external applications/actuators through which the user is able to interact actively without using the usual physiological pathways of peripheral nerves and muscles. Despite the fact that this technology is still at an experimental stage and in any case is limited to clinical environments, there has been increased interest in bringing BCI into the daily lives of users. Various European projects have been started up aimed at reaching this objective. Even if this field of research is rich in ideas and implementations, there are still some question marks over methodology ethics, costs and stable engineering solutions for the large scale use of this technology.

As for *epimeleia,* I refer the reader to the analysis of what Bellingreri (2005, 2006) defines as pedagogical anthropology in an empathetic style, a perspective that, in line with what I developed in paragraph 4.2, aims for a philosophical vision of life and the world as a personal anamorphosis of the being. The universe is interpreted here as an immense educational device which can prepare the coming of a higher form of existence. A real educator's "educational love" is envisaged: they know how to offer themselves, to give of themselves without wanting to hold anything of themselves back. At this level, the phenomenological analysis takes empathy above all as a motivated act, one that is not spontaneous but conscious and free inasmuch as it the individual has a reason for performing this act. In this regard, what E. Stein (1917) wrote in *The Problem of Empathy* remains relevant, where the fact that empathy doesn't regard simply a gnoseological question but is of interest to the wider world of human communication, that is to say making sense of personal existence and of a community of people comes to light. Empathy as lived by the consciousness is not just a vital sentiment but a psychic act. Nevertheless, as opposed to psychology, phenomenology studies it as an intentional act, that is to say not solely a psychic act but a rational one (Armezzani et al., 2008). Amongst the intentional acts empathy is an original act that understands the other as the "you" of whose world my "I" has a part; just as conversely this "you" is part of my world. According to Stein, in the empathetic act, the other offers him or herself and is recognized as a "living body," inasmuch as he or she is a subject around whose gaze a world of objects and other subjects are arranged. Now, what the other lives and experiences is his or her "own" experience, which as such doesn't coincide with "my own experience." Therefore what is original for me is to feel that the other is living "their" feelings. I, for example, who cannot live the joy and the pain of the other, can however empathetically perceive that joy and that pain in my experience that includes what the other is living by placing myself in someone's position (Stein 1917). Thus the possibility of co-experiencing the world emerges, of having a common world through knowledge and empathic communication. This allows the integration of personal experiences of the world in a perspective that sees "that which is different" as a different way of understanding "that which is identical" (Callari Galli et al., 2005). Empathy in the end, in agreement with Bellingreri, opens up the possibility to live as a "we," to be a community. The other is understood as a you "for" another you, or as you "with" me. It is by virtue of this possibility that, at the same time empathy is revealed to be an essential experience for making sense of myself (Bellingreri, 2005, 2006).

In this situation, as Baccarini (2002, 2003) reveals, educating means taking care of the pupil; therefore the science of education can be interpreted as a supportive relationship, or better still, the science of care-giving. A science of the spirit, I would add, that can no longer be considered independent *tout court* of the organismic paradigm as proposed by the theory of complexity and then the bioeducational sciences. Subjects as subjects find themselves indeed on the other side of the subject–object dichotomy (Freeman, 2000b; Siegel, 1999; Fauenfelder, 2001). Nevertheless despite the synonymy of the body that presents itself to me, at the philosophical and anthropological level it is possible to observe a *plus:* the educational process in *sensu lato* should also take this excess of interiority, undeterminable objectively and phenomenologically, into account. Thus whoever teaches should care for the inner being of the spirituality of the subject in front of him (or better still with their original significance). In the therapeutic gesture, therefore, something is communicated which is beyond verbal language: between the two faces whose gaze meets, something happens that is not reducible to an informational measure, something which refers us to something else, to a significance whose revelation (or transmission) is already a dissimulation in the continual process of incarnation of intentionality at the level of the monad minds. It seems clear therefore at this point that the educational crisis corresponds to an anthropological crisis and that crisis coincides with a crisis of meaning understood as direction (in what direction should I go?) and significance (who am I?), that is to say, total disorientation.

The orientation, the direction to follow that is indivisibly tied to the project of being human should be supplied by education's filling the spiritual dimension of man with sense. In the Greek definition of man as a spiritual being his *telos* is indeed already inscribed. In truth the term "spiritual" implies a tension between the absolute which transcends the empirical (the organismic dimension understood as a dialectic synthesis or systemic unity of *bios* and *psyche*) and that has been, in my opinion, explored magisterially by the Austrian psychiatrist Frankl (1972) who in *Ten Theses of the Person*, a short but intense work in which the value and sense of human existence shines through, writes:

> man as a person is not a factual being but a facultative being, he exists in agreement with his possibilities in favor of which or against which he can decide. That is why Jaspers has defined man as a being that decides. And as a being that decides, he is diametrically opposed to what psychoanalysis affirms, which emphasizes is the 'being pushed.' Being a man is above all a deep and radical *being responsible.* Which is to say that he is more than just a free being: in responsibility man's liberty is defined, that is to say, man is free inasmuch as he decides for or against. [. . .] The person is not determined by his impulses but oriented in a direction. Whilst from the psychoanalytical perspective the person aspires to pleasure, in the optic of existential analysis this points to values. (Frankl, 1972, p. 111).

The liberty that makes up the person's own dimension is in fact, according to the father of speech therapy, the response to someone or something; authentic life is the moment when a person fully realizes him- or herself, recognizing that human existence is guided by a desire for meaning. This person can be unconscious but that mysterious dimension now assumes a new face: in the unconscious the spiritual sinks its roots. The source of the person in Frankl's eyes represents the spiritual reality of man, a place of liberty and the revelation of transcendence. From this point of view then, the idea of person completes, by questioning from within its own scientific investigation, the utilitarian concept that the person is reduced exclusively to organism, that is to say the ensemble of organs (instruments) that are limited to carrying out specific functions. The person, in agreement with Frankl is to be found beyond the psycho-physical organism: he is subtle. The spiritual persona sustains the organism but needs it to express itself and act.[4] Thus the organism is a means to an end: the realization of human dignity. For the Austrian psychiatrist:

> The person establishes the psycho-physico-spiritual complex, which represents man's essence. We only know the spiritual person in coexistence with its psychic-physical organism. Man, therefore, represents a point of intersection, a crossroads of the three levels of existence: the physical, the psychic and

> the spiritual. These levels of existence cannot be separated from each other [. . .] it would be false therefore to affirm that man is made up of the physical, psychic and spiritual. He is in fact a unified whole" (p. 113).

In light of all this, then, at the philosophical level it is possible to infer that no educational project can avoid having as an objective the specific form of the human person, a development, that is, that does not overlook his essence (*eidos*): realizing what is already man's constitutional and structural nature (Gervilla, 2000; Jimenz Rios, 2000). In this sense the concept of form and the dynamic processes of growth is what bioeducational research is most interested in and can be evidenced in the form of thought. Thought, indeed, in our opinion is not just a biological mechanism, genetic potential, but is also, and above all, intentionality incarnated in human symbolic language, thus creating ever new meanings.

> All of this brings us to a radical redefinition of the concept of adaptation which, in the traditional definition, considered the environment as the origin of changes to the system; under this meaning the input-output model is dominant and adaptation is defined as a response of the system to environmental needs. According to this new meaning, the conservation of the system, that is to say the conservation of the life cycles that define its organization, become of primary importance. It is interesting to note that in this light the logic of an evolutionism that is tied to the environment is so little expressed as to place in crisis the very concept of isomorphism that links species and the environment to a harmonic synchronism (Frauenfelder, 2004, p. 90).

Indeed, these considerations lead us again to Varela's key hypothesis (1979) regarding the characteristics of living systems, namely, the idea that these are autopoietic systems, in other words, that they are able to produce their own identity. Consequently, autopoietic systems, even if they are materially modified, are autonomous in the sense that they subordinate every change to the maintenance of their own organization (Maturana, Varela, 1980). This progressive maturation of the idea of autonomy and organizational closure by biological research is an extremely interesting aspect of contemporary scientific research which currently is moving the reflection on form towards formulations that go from the world of structure to the hypothetic potentials of the DNA code in its deep information (semantic aspect of *bios*) (Di Bernardo, 2012). In this sense a behavior that takes form is always tied to a biological characteristic (the plasticity of the nervous system), but it is only realized in function of an experience in contact with the environment and in any case is not determined by genetics (Di Bernardo, 2010). Even this last interpretation recognizes the foreign, the other-than-self in educational processes. Thus the comparison between the neurosciences and philosophy and anthropology in educational contexts is one of the most important challenges that the bioeducational sciences will have to face in relation to the biodynamic perspective (Santoianni, 1998; Santoianni, Striano, Frauenfelder 2000; Frauenfelder et al., 2004), a perspective, that is, that on the basis of the new paradigm linked to the science of complexity shows the need today to refer to a new circularity that is capable of bringing a philosophy that is discovering in ever greater depth the role of analysis in the great questions about the meaning of life nearer to science which in turn is thankfully becoming aware of the need to not let the deep questions concerning significance and intentionality fall by the wayside.

4.4 Functional realism and knowledge construction

After having shown, based on contemporary complexity theory and the latest research in the field of neuroscience, removal from the original computational matrix that orients the current studies on the functionalities of the cognitive constitutes a real challenge for the mind science. It is a challenge that induces one to think again in an interdisciplinary, systemic and evolutive way about the problem of knowledge: we need an approach that is able to hold together, while at the same time keeping distinct, the various levels of reference, the holism of the sciences of the spirit, and the methodological reductionism proper to the natural sciences. Therefore, from this viewpoint, these conclusive paragraphs center on identifying an epistemological framework capable of realizing the synthesis just mentioned, making reference to autopoietic systems, the theory of the auto-organization, genetic epistemology, the cognitive activities of molecular biology, the biology of meaning, and neurophenomenology.

The topic of cognition is faced, then, by a new paradigm capable of bringing together knowledge objectivity and the functional plasticity proper of the living systems. In this sense, the studies done by Maturana and Varela concerning the relationship, at a biological level, between cognition and auto-organization are pioneering, as are the studies done by Kandel for what concerns synaptic plasticity and distributed memory, Carsetti's investigation at a level of non-standard semantics and, finally, the latest attempts to identify measures of information (biological information) able to go beyond statistical rarity and computational incompressibility.

The definition of a multisystemic concept of memory substantiated by advances in neuroscience seems to have led epistemological studies to consider with growing interest the cognitive nature of the subject and the plurality of factors of mnestic processes (Gardner, 1991; Sternberg, Grigorenko, 1997) with the goal of focusing on and bringing attention to the diversity of learning stimuli offered and how, in function of these, the way a pupil processes memories tends to vary (Santoianni, 2006; Santoianni, Striano, 2003). Memory, like knowledge is therefore profoundly "situated" and "distributed" in the memories shared within a socio-cultural system (environmental meaning) and intersubjective relationships, that are shown to be essential for the construction and transmission of mnestic products considered as a "platform of shareable and transferable references" (Santoianni, Striano, 2000).

Although it is divided into areas that are probably specifically "entrusted" with performing mnestic functions, the entire brain as a dynamic non-linear system is involved in recuperating memories; yet, despite Kandel's promising research, it is still unclear how these memories are located and how they are preserved (Salomon, 1993). In general, however, memory is a process that is epigenetically characterized and that depends on the growth of the nervous system (Jablonka, Lamb 2005; Keller, 2003, 2010) and is linked to the ensemble of the person and his cognitive system: from perceptive processes to superior mental processes, bringing into play various elements from affectivity to motivational components, from modes of cognitive configuration to thought processing organization (Bruner, 1983, 1993; Sabatano 2005). In this sense the concept of form can be described as a dynamic process of growth, and the concept of form which especially concerns psychogenetic investigation, can be seen as the "form of thought" or *Forma formans.*

Thought, according to the perspective explained in these pages, is not only a biological mechanism or genetic potential, but also a precise dialectic process in which the form of environmental stimulation conditions and makes this potential concrete through a couple of selections (internal and external) in determined directions. The energy and information that an organism obtains exploring the external world reflect the reality specifically linked to its own way of responding to the changed environmental situations. Thought, in other words, it is to be understood, in my opinion, especially as intentionality that embodies itself in symbolic human language, creating new meanings. Symbolic forms that permit a growth of the entire being of the knowing subject of a system circularity where the observer and the source co-evolve continuously as they are parts of a process of knowledge's growth. Maturana and Varela (1980, 1992) distinguish, in this regard, the subject matter of biology (an organism's functioning) from the cognitive processes of the biological entity (the description of its behavior and its relations with the environment and with other systems). These aspects correspond to the observation of a living system in two different and complementary perspectives: from an internal point of view placed inside the dynamic system, the organism's relationships with its environment are irrelevant, while from the external point of view we can distinguish between what is a system and what is defined as environment. At this second level, what disappears is the meaning of the dynamics within the system itself, which thus comes to be characterized by complementary properties of openness (proper to the particular system structure) and closeness (proper to the entity's organization), each in turn defined by the interpretation of the concepts of "organization" and "structure" (Maturana, Varela, 1980). In this sense, a system's organization is the result of the relations between its components that must remain invariant for it to retain its identity. A system's structure, on the other hand, is defined as that particular set of components and of relations through which the system's organization is made manifest in a particular environment inasmuch as it is a specific spatio-temporal entity (Frauenfelder, 2001). The relation between these two properties make it possible to distinguish the living being and the environment as elements independent from each other, among which, a necessary structural congruence can be observed (Maturana, Varela, 1973), within which a disturbing agent (the environment) triggers an effect that is determined by the structure of the being disturbed—the living being, that with its structure determines its own change in relation to the disturbance (Varela et al., 1991; Varela, 1997). These reflections lead to a deep redefinition of the key concept of adaptation, surpassing the classical definition which considered the environment the origin of the system changes (at this level, adaptation is simply the system's response to the environment's inputs) in function of a predominant role played by the conservation of the system's autonomy, understood as maintenance of the autopoietic cycles that define its organization (self-organized criticality) (Varela et al. 1999; Kauffman 1993, 2000).

We thus find ourselves, at the evolutionary level, facing a dynamic situation that becomes and transforms itself through successive equilibria. On the one hand, the necessary preservation of stability in replication entails eliminating a variety of noise pathways. This expulsion, from the identical island of replication, of openness and underlying tension, of random internal and external aggressions, constitutes an objective impoverishment of the expressive capacity in terms of growth and of revelation in the profound sense of the structure that is reproduced. On the other hand, the creative use of random shifts, the ordered inclusion of mutations allow for a real growth of an entity's structures (Carsetti, 1987, 2000b). But this usage cannot be increased beyond a certain threshold without the structure losing its own identity, its own characteristics of internal stability, unitary and balanced control of a process that reveals itself in pathways always more branched and differentiated. Therefore, the identity is no longer construed restrictively, as simple, i.e., as surface identity. The invariance, in fact, that should be protected in a development situation is that relating to the unitary coordination of profound patterns of growth (Carsetti, 1999). It is precisely within this dynamic relationship between surface and depth, according to Carsetti, that we can find the *telos* able to reveal to us how it is possible to maintain an identity of an analytical nature, despite the progressive and synthetic transformation of the informational structures (Carsetti, 2005b). It then seems plausible to think that, precisely within the folds of this intrinsic connection lies the origin, at least for certain aspects, of the metamorphoses of nature *(Natura naturata),* one of the reasons that drive the continual emergence of the new (Carsetti, 2000b; Varela, 1983, 1999).

The main thesis provided by Varela is that living beings are autopoietic systems, capable, that is, of building themselves producing, therefore, their own identity. Thus, these systems, even if they concretely modify themselves, are autonomous, as they subordinate every change to maintaining their own organization (Varela, 1979). This evolution of the idea of autonomy and of organization by the life sciences represents a fundamental aspect of the contemporary scientific context (Kauffman, 2008), which is expecting a shift in its reflections on "form" (Atlan, 1995) towards the passage by the real of the given structures to the realm of the infinitary capabilities (from an informational point of view) of the DNA code (Gabora et al, 2013; Blasone, Vitiello, 2011). Maturana (1978, 1997, 2007) and Varela (1983, 1997) have intuited with great acumen that, from a biological point of view, cognition is a process dependent upon the subject, and being a process, is also constitutive of the organization of the knowing subject. The scholars have evidenced that cognition is subordinated to the autopoiesis of the knowing subject itself, highlighting, at the same time, the close relationship that occurs between cognition and life: being and knowing, in fact, are reciprocally conditioned. In this sense, according to Kandel (2001, 2005), a behavior that takes shape is always linked to a biological feature (synaptic plasticity), but occurs only in relation to experience, through contact with the environment and, in any case, is not determined by the "genetic program" (Di Bernardo 2007, 2011). The epistemological discourse may then refer to two different parameters of connection with the external stimulus. In first place, the neo-evolutionary adaptation conceives the input as the possibility for the subject to explicate its own adaptive forces incidental to the plasticity of the human genetic makeup through the capability of the subject to adequate itself to the situations of stimulus that it faces during its development. So, the outside, by stimulating in the relationship above all an adaptive force, influences the construction of knowledge with a thrust of a qualitative (semantic) type, though one which is closely linked to the input, and therefore in some way dependent upon it (Maturana, Varela, 1980; Frauenfelder, 2001). In second place, the input perceived as disruption provokes in the subject the realization of an autopoietic restructuring through the resorting to a coupled process of assimilation and canalization capable of guiding the ontogenesis (Waddington, 1966). Thus, the input seen as disruption triggers an autopoietic defense process which responds to the input by renovating its subjectivity in its entirety (Maturana, Varela, 1980). In this process where a proper subjectivity is unveiled that is maintained under the form of a coagulum, the output arises as a product of the biological subject itself. In this guise, it is possible to glimpse at the horizon of these reflections the possibility to interpret the outside, which is, however, the cause of the disruption, as an assimilated and canalized stimulus (*adaequatio*) through complex and highly-sophisticated processes, surely much more intricate than adaptive operation understood in a classical sense, ascribable to a linear kind of description (standard models). These two different coupling strategies (Maturana, Varela, 1980, 1992) with the outside express, within a deep process of form production through a continuous creative action of cutting out symbolic forms (formation of thought), and, therefore, of a dynamic process of growth of knowledge, different epistemological implications and suggestions (Piaget, 1971, 1973).

Within such a framework, it should also be noted that at the level of a biological organism, just as with an integrated communication system that reaches a certain level of complexity, the reality we experience daily, when we are dealing with phenomena of flow and the recording of information, is characterized by the constant existence of "channel-level noise" and by the close connection of a circular nature that exists between the recording activity at the sensory level and observation activities at the intellectual level. As we implied in the third chapter, making reference to some of Carsetti's works, the detection of the continuous presence of these two essential conditions leads us to postulate the existence, within the source, of a displacement of information according to orders of increasing depth, or subsequent stages of complexity that must be gradually explained and brought to the surface. Essential in this design is the role of noise, understood as a clue to new forms of organization, as well as the supporting framework for the deployment of renewed mediation schemes able to lay the conditions for a better integration between the observer and the source: when it acts on the signal, in fact, the amount of output information increases because at the same time the uncertainty grows. Noise, therefore, can help reveal a hidden type of information, a fabric of rules that determines the evolution of the system from within. Through noise there come to us, albeit in a concealed way, instructions concerning the interplay of possibilities, clues that guide the selective imagination to discover new worlds. We must keep in mind, in regard to this, the relevant research provided by Freeman in the field of neurodynamics and the precious help given by the technique of neuroimaging, able to disclose the mysterious world of brain activities of non-conscious subjects. However, such clues will be significant for us only to the extent that we can assimilate them, weaving, moreover, in function of them, a more complex and deeper explanation of our development. In this framework, the epigenetic structures alive at the sensory level then appear to be filters in the making whose growth is guided indirectly by the intellect through successive changes in the design of measurements, at the probabilistic and relational level, obtained through recourse to specific reflection procedures and specific methodical instruments (Carsetti, 2012a).

If at the level of reflection, within the framework of the outline that is proposed here, one has a transformation that privileges the categorical associative moment, through the abstraction and purification of encoding and synthesis operations of the information provided, at the level of knowledge, the system should work on symbolic representations in itself, on knowledge as "internalized forms." At this stage, according to Carsetti (1999, 2000a, 2000b), there would be no pre-given synthesis modules, but guidelines capable of designing an area renewed by the invention and selection of new cognitive tools. We thus find ourselves not before an automaton with pre-programmed finite states (as in the Monodian model), but before a generative language (DNA is a complex system of an infinitary nature able to grow and change as a result of displacement and becoming of transposable elements, albeit in compliance with the basic conditions for the entity's coordination and its internal functioning) with partial abilities to self-program endowed, within the entity, with control and self-regulation centers. In this sense, we can assume, in agreement with Carsetti (2004), that it is this intricate path that allows, at least in part, to come to some sort of assimilation, indirectly, of the external message, an assimilation that strengthens the connection between the environment and the internal self-organizational processes. That could lead, as it has been pointed out above, to the birth of connections that are multidimensional, typical of the stratified logic that characterizes, at the embryonic level, the development of a living system. Only after this will we have the phenomena of selection and stabilization (Carsetti, 1984a, 1984b). And in fact, as was already clear to Waddington more than sixty years ago, if the external compression blocks the expression of certain genes, the generative process that characterizes the system will be forced to find new trajectories and new paths, to look for possible arrangements to preserve the background conditions of its own internal consistency (Waddington, 1957, 1966; Kandel, 1993). As we have seen in the third chapter, therefore, in the context of the information theory it currently seems to be widely accepted both that the programs written in the direct morphogenesis of genetic memory, and that the inscription in memory, is morphogenesis in act (Omodeo, 1984; Carsetti, 2005b). The wealth of memories that forms the most intimate part of every man, and serves also as an important behavioral basis for each animal, is constituted through the brain's physical transformation, albeit at a level that only in these last few years has been possible to detect using functional neuroimaging techniques, but not yet to measure fully at the strictly qualitative level.[5]

There opens, thus, a chapter of research, at once new and old,[6] that represents one of the fulcrums of the ongoing investigation at the level of the epistemological and cognitive sciences (Carsetti, 2004). By virtue of the discoveries we have made during the journey so far undertaken, it seems we may safely affirm, with Carsetti, that:

> Cognitive activity is rooted in reality, but at the same time represents the necessary means whereby reality can

> embody itself in an objective way: in accordance with an in-depth nesting process and a surface unfolding of operational meaning. In this sense, the objectivity of reality is also proportionate to the autonomy reached by cognitive processes. Within this conceptual framework, reference procedures thus appear as related to the modalities providing the successful constitution of the channel, of the actual link between operations of vision and thought. Such procedures ensure not only a 'regimentation' or an adequate replica, but, on the contrary, the real constitution of a cognitive autonomy in accordance with the truth (Carsetti, 2013, p. 104).

The role of cognitive procedures, therefore, is to guide the primary informational streams and the selective forces involved, which arise as effective instruments for the continuous renewal of the code, for the emergence of ever new incompressibility. Hence the ability to define new axiomatic systems, as well as the real development of continuous reconstruction processes at the semantic level (Carsetti, 2013). It is, in fact, only by a complete "reduction" at the level of the first order and a non-standard analysis at the level of the higher orders, that new incompressibility will come to develop on the effective level. In other words, through an adequate theory of natural information it is possible to insert into the same epistemological framework Kandel's methodological reductionism (the molecular biology of cognitive activities) on one hand and the systemic approach proper to intentional complexity (Freeman's neurodynamics), on the other hand, in order to delineate new paradigms which favor a continuous growth of knowledge. Whence the concrete possibility of a connection between the things you see and the things you do not see, between identifying something visually and the thoughts regarding the connections that exist between such things (the proper task of the philosophy of science which does not want to reduce itself, following the line of Popper, to mere languistic analysis) (Husserl, 1900, 1901, 1939). Behold, therefore, emerge the linkage between the eyes of the mind with the eyes of meaning, a meaning that makes itself generativity and thought. In the article entitled "Functional realism, non-standard semantics and the genesis of the mind's eyes," Carsetti writes about this matter:

> Meaning can selectively express itself only through a) the nested realization, at the abstract level, of specific 'fusion' processes, b) the determination of specific schemes of coherence able to support this kind of realization, c) a more and more cooperative and unified articulation at the deep level of the primary informational fluxes, d) the identification of a model able to reflect and renew within itself as a fixed point the original meaning 'word.' It shapes the forms in accordance with *Sinn* connections, precise stability factors, symmetry choices, coherent contractions and ramified completions. We can partially inspect (and 'feel') this kind of embodiment, at the level, for instance, of 'categorial intuition,' insofar as we successfully manage to reconstruct, identify and connect the attractors of this particular dynamic process. It is exactly by means of the successive identification and guided *compositio* of these varying attractors that we can manage to imprison the thread of meaning and identify the coherent and becoming texture of the constraints concerning the architecture of visual thinking. In this way we shall finally be able to obtain a first self-representation of our mental activities, thus realizing a form of effective autonomy: a representation that exactly concerns the «narration» relative to the progressive opening of the eyes of our mind and the correlated constitution of the *Cogito* and its rules (Carsetti, 2006, p. 178).

According to this perspective, therefore, at the level of intuition-based categorization processes, the original meaning is renewed through the production of ever-new forms. The processes of unification of forms, carried out on the conceptual level as a result of the file's registration (a file selected by the morphogenesis in act), develop thus as modules, as attractors operating at the level of connective forms and that arise as multiplication factors at the internal level (Carsetti, 2005a). Behold, then, the possibility of having natural forms animated by an internal code, which are created over time with reference to operations inscribed in a project. It is, in other words, an autonomous and selective production of forms that, once modulated according to concepts, becomes vision on the basis of principles. An original meaning will, then, at the same time multiply and unify itself over time as a process unfolding within the context of a specific production of natural forms:

> With respect to this frame of reference, Reality presents itself as a set of becoming processes characterized by the presence-irradiation of a specific body of meaning and by an inner (iterative) *compositio* of generative fluxes having an original character. These processes then gradually articulate through and in a (partially-consistent) unifying development warp with internal fluctuations of functional patterns. [. . .] Only the individual capable of representing and tuning the work as living harmony, and the score as silent object, will actually be able to depict him/her self as 'I' and as subject. [. . .] The 'thinking I' which surfaces and the meaning which emerges thus fuse in the expression of a work which ultimately manages to articulate and unite itself with the awareness-*Cogito* and the ongoing narration: an observer thus joins a work acting as a filigree. [. . .] not a simple gestaltic restructuring, but the growth and multiplication of cognitive processes and units, i.e. the actual regeneration and multiplication of original Source according to the truth (Carsetti, 2006, pp. 191–193).

According to this point of view the selection and partial internal transformation of the models, of the individual paths "in the maze of alter nativity," depend on the last level, from an objective point of view, of the evolution and final landing point of a complicated process of a paired nature that sees the reciprocal interaction between observer and reality (a reality which, according to Carsetti, constitutes and interweaves from within the biological and cognitive fibers of the observer himself) and which also sees, as a final result, the emergence of a metamorphosis that is connected to the subsequent revelation of nuclei of depth information, as well as the emergence of specific forms of creativity which are the counterpart to "the discovery and awareness of new ways-realizations of truth" (Carsetti, 1991), a truth that, according to Mittelstaedt (1990), at the level of statements, will not be absolute, but relative to the manner in which it is given. This manner does not refer only to the relationship with a given world—and to the presentation of this world to the intellect—but to a collection of interactive processes of observing, measuring and processing information (truth as a dynamic relationship, as an unfolding process of deep meaning). A world thus, in agreement with Carsetti, appears to us, on the one hand, as a correlation of functions and, on the other hand, as the result of specific processes of interference between systems-worlds: correlation and product connected from time to time to specific properties of self-reflection and forms of structural coupling with an observer (Carsetti, 1991). At this level, then, the truth is not understood as simple correspondence, but as emergence of the new states of consistency, balance and stabilization (Carsetti, 1991; Vitiello, 2009a, 2009b). Truth as a "form of constraint" and as "a changeable fabric of selection" (Carsetti, 1988, 1999) that is later discovered, and that reflects itself inasmuch as it is correspondence, only when the stabilization itself is reached in an objective manner (*adaequatio*). Such correspondence, therefore, appears as mediated by the measures and processes of informational elaboration that come to be implemented (truth as assimilation, cognition and life) and it can be defined, from an operational and scientifical point of view, only in relation to such processes[7].

In light of all this, therefore, the study of the mechanisms of information transmission today needs new measures of complexity, measures (new axiomatic systems), namely, that must not address only statistical rarity (Shannon, 1948) or computational incompressibility (Kolmogorov, 1965; Chaitin, 1974, 1987), but should also be able to take into account the coupled connection between the source and the living (or cognitive) agent, the evolution of this connection, and the subsequent constitution of real processes of continuous reorganization at the semantic level (Carsetti, 2013). For example, we will no longer be able to speak of individuals, of a given domain of individuals etc., but of functions and fixed points within a set of functional transformations (Carsetti, 2000a, 2000b, 2004). In this guise, complexity is not simply related to a given sequence, but will be related to something that is detected with difficulty and which opens up within itself also in virtue of the modalities through which the process of exploration gradually manages to express itself. The observer's skill in creating his own measures comes, therefore, to form an intrinsic part of the given object or fact's very process of constituting itself as given for the observer. In this way, at the epigenetic level, memory, and meaningful complexity are closely connected to the realization, diachronically, of a holistic process that can only be characterized in terms of a higher-order logic (morphogenesis in act), a process inside of which the relation of alternatives between systems and worlds manifests itself as the product of specific interference patterns within which is located the origin of the teleonomical articulation characterizing the process itself (Carsetti, 2005b). The mnestic function configures itself, therefore, as a dynamic and profound process that reconstructs and connects operations of internal self-reflection, rather than as one that simply "stores" data in a static mental space. Just like the world of the first monadic order, in which Shannon's classic measure of information has pride of place, it appears linked to the existence of forms of invariance and to the defining of univocal spaces of measurement; at the higher-order levels, instead (though already at the polyadic level) we have the presence of specific dichotomies, of different potentials that present themselves simultaneously, of alternative measurements, of an evolutionary bricolage that is carried out through successively interlocking states yet which are bound together in a holistic way (Carsetti, 2010a). In fact, at the level of a biological system of information processing we find ourselves before a system that is essentially characterized by the fact that what is self-organizing within itself is the very function that determines such information along with its meaning (Atlan, 2000). But it is precisely to the extent that the system constitutes itself as an autonomous reality that the origin of the meaning regarding the self-organization of the system manages to reveal itself (organicity), on the objective level, as an emergent property (Carsetti, 1999, 2000a). And it is at this precise point that we can recognize that particular entanglement of complexity, self-organization, intentionality and emergence that characterizes the natural forms of human mnemonic activity.

NOTES

Notes to Chapter 1

1. In the sense that the mind is shared, distributed and embedded; yet not for this reason can the mind's expressive power ever be considered separately from the brain. See for more information: E. Frauenfelder and F. Santoianni, *Nuove frontiere della ricerca pedagogica tra bioscienze e cibernetica* (Napoli: Edizioni Scientifiche Italiane, 1997).

2. The second chapter discusses the molecular and cognitive mechanisms of memory, while part of the third chapter is devoted to studying biological information from an epistemological point of view.

3. Recently, the *European Task Force on Disorders of Consciousness* (2010) proposed replacing VS with a less catchy, but more descriptive term: *Unresponsive Wakefulness Syndrome* (UWS), (Laureys *et al.*, 2010). Cf. S. Laureys et al.,"Consciousness, Unresponsive wakefulness syndrome: a new name for the vegetative state or apallic syndrome," *BMC Med* 8 (2010): 68. The term *unresponsive* was chosen to indicate that patients manifest reflex activity but are unresponsive to commands. *Wakefulness* refers to the opening of the patient's eyes (whether spontaneous or stimulus-induced)—something never observed in coma. *Syndrome* underlines the fact that we are considering a number of clinical factors.

4. Despite the British Royal College of Physicians (2003) having redefined the diagnostic criteria for VS in its guidelines, evidence has begun to accumulate of a high incidence of diagnostic errors, reaching percentages as high as 43% and for this reason an "implementation of the guidelines is likely to require significant investment in rehabilitation services."

5. The diagnostic distinction between VS and MCS, however, as a recent study by Schnakers showed, has not significantly reduced the risk of diagnostic error in current clinical practice, inasmuch as the rate of misdiagnosis of VS is still about 41%, while MCS is wrongly diagnosed in about 10% of cases. Cf. C. Schnakers et al., "Diagnostic accuracy of the vegetative and minimally conscious state: clinical consensus versus standardized neurobehavioral assessment," *BMC Neurology* 21 (2009): 9–35.

6. The nosographic category of MCS includes some forms (at least two) of akinetic mutism syndrome. This syndrome is often confused with VS. Patients with akinetic mutism appear wakeful and attentive but remain immobile while maintaining the ability to follow movements through *smooth pursuit* (slow visual tracking). This clinical sign observed in akinetic mutism is absent in VS. Cf. B. Jennet and M. Bond, "Assessment of outcome after severe brain injury," *Lancet* 1 (1975): 480–484.

7. Patients with this syndrome, which is caused by pontine damage, respond in the initial phase after injury in a manner similar to patients in MCS. Precisely because of the peculiar characteristics of this pathology, misdiagnosis can occur, sometimes with serious consequences (e.g., suspension of care) and improper behavior by physicians in the absence of thoroughly informed consent.

8. This study was based on the observation that states that can be seen as forms of self-consciousness occur even in the absence of relations with the external world, as in alert wakefulness or in dreams. It was found that these states are often associated with the ability of specialized cortical areas to interact and an efficient technique has been developed—that we will study in the next paragraph—to gauge the presence of such interactive activities. This research made waves in numerous media outlets, which proclaimed that it was finally possible to "measure consciousness." What had been developed, instead, was a technique for measuring the interactive activities between brain areas. To call such activities consciousness is to make an assertion lacking in any theoretical foundation. The definition of consciousness, indeed, remains totally open; this is even more true of its "minimum status."

9. The term 'Functional Neuroimaging' refers to the use of neuroimaging technologies that can measure brain metabolism in order to analyse and study the relationship between the activity of specific brain areas and specific brain functions. It is a tool of prime importance in cognitive neuroscience and neuropsychology. In addition to classic applications of experimental research to neurocognitive processes, functional neuroimaging techniques are becoming increasingly important in clinical and neurological diagnostics for the study of changes in the brain after traumatic, oncological, vascular and neurodegenerative pathologies. The most commonly used methods include positron emission tomography (PET), functional magnetic resonance imaging (fMRI), the multi-channel electroencephalogram (EEG), SPECT, magneto encephalography (MEG) and near-infrared spectroscopy (NIRS).

10. Changes in neural activity in the brain are associated with changes in energy demands: the greater the functional activity of a brain region, the higher its metabolism, and consequently, the higher its energy demands. One of the most sophisticated non-invasive techniques that exploit the hemodynamic changes produced by neuronal activity to identify the activated areas of the brain is functional magnetic resonance imaging (fMRI). This method of investigation is based on the change in the MRI signal, following a metabolic and hemodynamic response in a region where neuronal activation is induced by internal or external stimuli. The purpose of magnetic resonance imaging (MRI) is to obtain detailed images of the brain's anatomy by exploiting the nuclear properties of certain atoms in the presence of magnetic fields. Through data collection techniques, it is possible

to capture images that can follow and visualise the development of some metabolic phenomena. Using this methodology, one can: display changes of oxygenation in the cortical regions and reconstruct the map of brain activation during sensory, mental and motor functioning, with high spatial resolution.

11. An important contribution to the study of perception and of mechanisms integrating cerebral functioning in patients with disorders of consciousness (DOC) was furnished by data from drug-induced comas on volunteers undergoing general anaesthesia. Both populations show a similar behavior consisting of residual activation, in response to external stimuli, of segregated cortical islands that include the trunk, the thalamus and the primary low-level cortices. But it is precisely in the manner of this residual activation that a functional factor has been discovered that differentiates VS from MCS. In VS patients as well as in those under anaesthesia, one observes no activation of higher-level areas including the frontoparietal and median networks. In contrast, patients in MCS can manifest an activation of high-level areas, just like the control subjects (Doble *et al.*, 2003). Cf. J.E. Doble et al., "Impairment, activity, participation, life satisfaction, and survival in persons with *locked-in* syndrome for over a decade: follow-up on a previously reported cohort," *J Head Trauma Rehabil* 18 (2003): 435–444.

12. Recent studies based on electrophysiological data and functional neuroimaging have shown that VS can be interpreted on a functional basis as a syndrome involving a disconnection between the cortical and cortico-thalamic areas; these studies furthermore show that some clinical patients in VS, in as much as 38% of cases, may have preserved a greater degree of connectivity, such as to allow even complex forms of processing environmental stimuli, but which can be recognized only with the help of precise instrumental tests Cf. P.V. Schoenle et al. "How vegetative is the vegetative state? Preserved semantic processing in VS patients-evidence from N 400 event-related potentials," *NeuroRehabilitation* 19 (2004): 329–34.

13. It is necessary here to recall the important distinction between VS, whether persistent or not, and brain death, which is perhaps not sufficiently clear to the public or even the media. Cf. J.B. Posner et al. "The neurophysiological bases of emotion: an fMRI study of the affective circumplex using emotion-denoting words," *Hum. Brain Mapp* 30 (2009): 883–895. What characterizes brain death is the presence of an irreversible coma, that is, an unresponsive coma associated with apnea, the absence of cephalic and spinal reflexes, and isoelectric EEG, all in the absence of drugs or hypothermia and lasting for at least 24 hours. No clinical analogy could ever be established between VS and brain death.

14. In the article entitled "Making Every Word Count for Nonresponsive Patients," Naci and Owen (August 12, 2013) show for the first time with

functional magnetic resonance imaging that behaviourally nonresponsive patients can use auditory selective attention to convey their ability to follow commands and communicate. One patient in a minimally conscious state was able to use attention to establish functional communication vis-à-vis the scanner, despite his inability to produce any communicative responses in repeated bedside examinations. More important, one patient, who had been in a vegetative state for 12 years before the scanning and remained in that state subsequent to it, was able to use his attention to correctly communicate answers to several binary questions. The technique may be useful in establishing basic communication with patients who appear unresponsive to bedside examinations and cannot respond with existing neuroimaging methods. Cf. L. Naci and A.M. Owen, "Making Every Word Count for Nonresponsive Patients," *Jama Neurol* (2013).

Notes to Chapter 2

1. In classical conditioning an animal learns to associate two events, for example the sound of a bell with the presence of food, so the animal begins to salivate as soon as it hears the sound of the bell, even in the absence of food. The animal has, in fact, learned that the sound of the bell precedes the arrival of food. In instrumental conditioning a living being will learn to associate proper behavior with a reward and wrong behavior with a punishment, so as to gradually change their behavior.

2. The founders of cognitive psychology, Bartlett, Tolman, Miller, Chomsky, Neisser, Simon and others, had difficulty in the early 1960s in convincing the scientific community of the limitations of behaviorism. These first cognitive psychologists, on the basis of studies by Gestalt psychologists, psychoanalysts and neurologists in Europe, sought to show that our knowledge of the world is based on our apparatuses responsible for perceiving the world, and that perception is a constructive process that depends not only on the information regarding the stimulus but also on the mental structure of the subject that processes it.

3. It was Wheeler, one of the leading theoretical physicists of the twentieth century at Princeton University, who formulated in 1990, for the first time, the idea that every physical body is ultimately composed of *energy* and *information*. This was expressed succinctly through his famous principle "it from bit." In other words, we say that every 'it'—every particle, every force field, even the very spatio-temporal continuum—derives its function, its meaning, its entire existence—though in some contexts only indirectly—from responses elicited from the apparatus to questions of a yes-no type, binary choices, 'bits.' "It from bit" captures the idea that each component of the physical world has deep down—very

deep, in the vast majority of cases—an *immaterial* source and explanation; what we call "reality" arises, ultimately, from asking "yes/no" questions and from recording responses evoked by from the apparatus" J.A. Wheeler, "Information, physics, quantum: The search for links," in *Complexity, entropy, and the physics of information,* ed. W. H. Zurek (Redwood City: Addison-Wesley, 1990), 75.

4. This interpretation is purely human (and thus at least hypothetically requires the presence of a human observer) and not intrinsic to the computer itself, which is nothing more than a physical signal processing device, devoid of any kind of expectations.

5. As Pessa and Penna pointedly note, the classes of possible physical events, to which each symbol—identifying a particular representational state of mind—is associated, in practice, always consist of an infinite number of elements: this renders the link quite tenuous between the world of symbols—the world of mental processes—and the world of the physical processes corresponding to them. All this creates numerous difficulties for those who oppose reductionist positions and who, therefore, are engaged in the search for the neuro-physiological substrate of all the cognitive processes. Cf. M.P. Penna and E. Pessa, *Introduzione alla psicologia connessionista* (Roma: Di Renzo, 1998).

6. The psychologist Tulving was the first to propose the idea that explicit memory can be further subdivided into episodic memory—concerning events and personal experiences—and semantic memory—concerning the knowledge of facts and concepts. Cf. E. Tulving, "Episodic and semantic memory," in *Organization of memory,* eds. E. Tulving and W. Donaldson (New York: Academic Press, 1972), 381–403.

7. The connectionist paradigm will be analyzed in the next chapter in relation to two concepts essential to continuing our discussion on the search to identify those elements at the basis of cognition, memory and identity: these concepts are information and meaning.

8. For example, when a person is asked a question, the concepts in the question "trigger" certain "nodes" of the semantic network representing the person's knowledge. This process of "activation" is propagated from one node to another, "spreading activation," and allows one to obtain an answer either by activating new nodes, different from those originally activated, or through the identification of the nodes where activation processes from different starting points converge.

9. H. M. was a 27-year-old man who had suffered from bilateral epileptic seizures of the temporal lobe, resistant to any treatment, which were the result of a brain injury suffered at age 9. A surgical operation was performed to remove bilaterally from his brain the hippocampus, amygdala, and parts of the multimodal associative areas of the temporal lobe. After surgery, the

removal of the medial temporal lobe part resulted in the emergence of a serious memory deficit: amnesia. H.M.'s short-term memory, on the order of seconds or a few minutes, was normal. He also retained a good long-term memory of events before the operation. Though expressing a certain degree of retrograde amnesia for the concepts acquired in the years just prior to the surgery. What H.M. now lacked totally was the ability to transfer new mnemonic traces from short-term to long-term memory. He was not able to remember for more than a minute any information about people, places or objects. For example, he had occasion to meet with Milner, but every time he saw her he acted as if he was seeing her for the first time. Cf. B. Milner et al., "Further analysis of the hippocampal amnesic syndrome: 14-year follow-up study of HM," *Neuropsychologia* 6 (1968): 215–234; E.R. Kandel, J.H. Schwartz and T.M. Jessell, *Principles of neural sciences,* 4th ed. (New York: The McGraw-Hill Companies, 2000).

10. H.M.'s case is not unique. All patients with extensive bilateral lesions of the limbic associative areas of the temporal lobe, whether due to surgeries or illness, have similar memory deficits.

11. Thanks to Milner's work, we now have reason to believe that concepts previously acquired are stored in the cerebral cortex, including the lateral temporal lobe, i.e., in those areas that initially processed the information. Cf. B. Milner, L.R. Squire and E.K. Kandel, "Cognitive Neuroscience and the Study of Memory," *Neuron,* 20 (1998): 445–468.

12. This concept is of paramount importance for current studies on post-genomics, focused on analysing the semantic aspects of the *bios.* Kandel's research, therefore, anticipates by a few decades the study of meaning and functions in biology both at the level of the genome (functional genomics) and at the level of proteins (Proteomics); the latter field of studies has exploded since 2000, subsequent to the early results from the sequencing of the human genome Cf. E. Fox Keller, *The Century of the Gene* (Cambridge: Harvard University Press, 2000); M. Di Bernardo, *Per una rivisitazione della dottrina monodiana della morfogenesi autonoma alla luce dei nuovi scenari aperti dalla post-genomica* (Roma: Aracne, 2007).

13. For example, we see a person's face rather than hearing their voice, because nerve cells in the eye's retina are linked with those portions of the brain (the visual system) that process and interpret visual information. For an in-depth analysis see: G. Edelman, *The Remembered Present: A Biological Theory of Consciousness* (New York: Basic Books, 1990); A. Carsetti, "Mental constructions and non-standard semantics," *La Nuova Critica* 33–34 (1999):101–126; Id., "Linguistic structures, cognitive functions and algebraic semantics," in *Functional models of cognition. Self-organizing dynamics and semantic structures in cognitive systems,* ed. Id. (Dordrecht: Kluwer, 2000a), 253–286.

14. A typical synapse is made up of three components: a presynaptic terminal, a postsynaptic target cell and a thin slit that separates the two neurons. This space, the *synaptic gap,* is about 20 nm wide (2 x 10^{-8} m). A cell's presynaptic terminal communicates through the synaptic gap with the cell body or dendrites of the postsynaptic target cell.

15. In the Fifties and Sixties, the British neurophysiologist Katz, in collaboration with other scholars, discovered that in presynaptic terminals the action potential induces the opening of membrane channels for calcium ions (Ca^{2+}). The opening of these channels, in turn, triggers a rapid and substantial increase in these same ions within the presynaptic terminals. This increase leads, finally, to the release of the neurotransmitter, which travels across the synaptic cleft and into the postsynaptic target cell. The interaction between the neurotransmitter and the receptors present on the postsynaptic cell causes depolarization in the postsynaptic membrane depolarization, resulting in the generation of an excitatory synaptic potential when this potential is high enough, and action potential is generated in the target cell. In a manner similar to the action potential, the synaptic potential is an electrical signal. Nonetheless, the two types of potentials are characterized by some substantial differences. While the action potential is a signal of considerable size, roughly 110 mV, the synaptic potential is far less strong and does not exceed a value ranging from 1mV to a few dozen millivolts. The value of the synaptic potential depends on a number of factors, including the number of presynaptic terminals activated and the amount of neurotransmitter able to reach the same postsynaptic cell. Cf. E.R. Kandel, *Cellular basis of behavior: an introduction to behavioral biology* (San Francisco: W. H. Freeman, 1976). In addition, the action potential exerts its function according to an "all-or-nothing" principle, while the synaptic potential is graduated and its amplitude depends on the number of molecules of neurotransmitter released from the presynaptic neuron and the number of receptors present in the postsynaptic cell able to bind the transmitter. Finally, the action potential is propagated actively: once created, it spreads without distortion from one end of the neuron to the other. Synaptic potential, however, propagates passively and if it is not high enough to generate an action potential, it decreases progressively along the neuron. Cf. L.R. Squire, "Memory and the hippocampus: a synthesis from findings with rats, monkeys, and humans," *Psychol. Rev.* 99 (2) (1992): 195–231; Id., "On the course of forgetting in very long-term memory," *Journal of Experimental Psychology: Learning, Memory and Cognition* 15 (1989): 241–245; Squire and Kandel, *Memory: from mind to molecules*).

16. For a deeper treatment on the concept of molecular semantics closely connected to that of biological information and, in more generally, the language of life (at the biochemical level) understood as an emergent

process whose rules (invariance) are the result of the coupled interplay of complex depth dynamics in continual evolution. Cf. H. Atlan, "Self creation of meaning," *Phys. Scr.* 36 (1987): 563–76; Id., "Intentional self-organization. Emergence and reduction. Towards a physical theory of intentionality," *Thesis Eleven* 52 (1998): 5–34; M. Di Bernardo, "Verso una fondazione naturalistica delle pre-condizioni dell'etica: semantica molecolare ed intenzionalità nei sistemi viventi," *Dialegesthai. Rivista telematica di filosofia,* (on line), a. XI.

17. Lashley, Köhler and other psychologists linked to Gestalt theory, for example, advanced the hypothesis that learning induced modifications in the electric fields or in the chemical gradients which they believed surrounded the populations of neurons and depended on the aggregate activity of the cells activated by the learning process. Alternatively, Forbes and de Nò suggested that memories were stored dynamically in self-stimulating neural circuits. Hebb later extended this idea in his theory of short-term memory. Finally Hyden advanced the hypothesis that learning induced changes in the basic composition of DNA or RNA. Cf. E.R. Kandel, "The Molecular Biology of Memory Storage: A Dialogue Between Genes and Synapses," *Science* 294 (5544) (2001): 1030–1038.

18. Kandel and collegues identified six motor neurons that establish direct connections with the respiratory organ and seven motor neurons that innervate the siphon. These latter neurons receive information directly (monosynaptically) from two related groups of about 40 sensory neurons that innervate the skin of the siphon. Sensory neurons, which release the neurotransmitter glutamate, are also linked to groups of excitatory and inhibitory interneurons, which in turn are projected towards the motor neurons. Stimulating the skin of the siphon thus triggers the sensory neurons, which directly trigger the motor neurons of the gill and siphon. Sensory neurons stimulate also different interneurons that, in turn, communicate with the motor neurons. The cells of this neuronal circuit are always the same, as are their interconnections. Thus, in every individual, a given cell is always connected to specific cells and not to others.

19. This discovery made by Kandel and his collegues was the first clear evidence of an evolutionary conservation of biochemical mechanisms between Aplysia and vertebrates.

20. The first clue of the importance of CREB in long-term memory was provided by Dash and Hochner—P.K. Dash, B. Hochner and E.K. Kandel, "Injection of cAMP-responsive element into the nucleus of Aplysia sensory neurons blocks long-term facilitation," *Nature* 345 (1990): 718–721. They injected oligonucleotides bearing the DNA element CRE, into the nucleus of a sensory neuron in culture, obtaining CREB through titring. This treatment prevents long-term facilitation, but not short-term. Afterwards Bartsch cloned CREB1-a in *Aplysia* (ApCREB-1a), showing that the injection

of the phosphorylated form of this transcription factor can in itself trigger the mechanism of long-term memory. Downstream of ApCREB Alberini and Bartsch discovered two positive transcription regulators, the protein that binds the CAAT sequence intensifier (ApC/EPB, CAAT box enhancer binding protein) and the activation factor (Ap/AF). Cf. C. Alberini et al. "C/EBP is a immediate-early gene required for the consolidation of long-term facilitation in Aplysia," *Cell.* 76 (1994): 1099–1114; D. Bartsch et al., "CREB-1 encodes a nuclear activator, a repressor, and cytoplasmic modulator that form a regulatory unit critical for long-term facilitation," *Cell* 95 (1998): 211–223 1998. CREB-1 activates on this set of genes, to immediate response: they in turn affect the genes downstream, thus resulting in the growth of new synaptic connections.

21. The first three types had already emerged, at least in part, from studies on learning and memory of which we presented a short summary in the previous paragraphs. The scientists Katz and Fatt inaugurated research in the realm of chemical transmission with the discovery of ionotropic receptors, or protein molecules that regulate the flow of ions through ion channels opened by neurotransmitters, producing a rapid synaptic action that lasts milliseconds. The next step was linked to the discovery of metabotropic receptors which activate second messenger pathways, such as the cAMP-PKA pathway, producing a slower synaptic activity, lasting minutes. As it was observed in *Aplysia,* this slow synaptic action can regulate the neurotransmitter release process, and therefore can contribute to the short-term memory of the sensitization. A third type of synaptic action, still more persistent (it can last days), derives from the repeated action of a neurotransmitter modulator such as serotonin. Cf. E. R. Kandel, "The Molecular Biology of Memory Storage: A Dialogue Between Genes and Synapses," *Science* 294 (5544) (2001): 1030–1038.

22. For a further development of Monodian research and, in particular, of the fundamental concepts of the gratuity of cellular processes and teleonomy see: V. Somenzi, *L'evoluzionismo* (Torino: Loescher, 1971); A. Carsetti, "Complessità e significato," in *Realismo, Semantica Formale e Teoria della Complessità,* Bologna, 1991, 1–20; Di Bernardo, *Per una rivisitazione della dottrina monodiana della morfogenesi autonoma;* Id., "Natural selection and self-organization in complex adaptive systems," *Rivista di Biologia / Biology Forum* 103 (1) (2010): 75–96; Id., *I sentieri evolutivi della complessità biologica nell'opera di S. A. Kauffman* (Milano: Mimesis, 2011).

23. An interesting example of the extent to which the memory depends on the environmental context comes from an experiment done on divers by Baddeley and Godden at the University of Cambridge. Cf. A.D. Baddeley, *Your Memory: A User's Guide* (New York: Firefly Books, 2004). Divers were made to listen to 40 unrelated words while on the beach or when they were

immersed in water at a depth of about 3 m. After learning, the divers had to remember as many words as they could while they were in one of two environmental contexts in which the learning had been carried out. The words memorized underwater were remembered better underwater, while the words stored on the beach were remembered better on the beach. Overall, divers remembered about 15% more words when the encoding and the recall took place in the same context. Although interesting, these effects should not be overestimated, since they seem to depend on the occurrence of rather substantial differences between the encoding and the evocation of the mood, mental status or the environment. These results emphasize, at any rate, the potential influence of recall stimuli. Cf. D.R. Godden and A.D. Baddeley, "Context-dependent memory in two natural environments: on land and underwater," *British Journal of Psychology* 66(3) (1975): 325–31; Squire, Kandel, *Memory: from mind to molecules.*

24. In some of the earliest works of this type, Fuster and colleagues (1997) taught primates to remember a color (the sample color) for about 16 seconds (delay period). At the end of this period of time they compared two or more colors and the animal was rewarded with juice if it selected the sample color. This exercise is called "delayed matching-to-sample." In the course of the experiment, Fuster recorded the activity of individual neurons in the TE area, an upper visual area located in the temporal lobe, believed to be important for the perception of visual objects. In this way, it was seen that many neurons in the TE area responded to the sample color when it appeared for the first time. It was particularly interesting to note that many neurons continued to respond even during the subsequent 16-second delay period, as if the persistent neural activity were a neuronal correlate of the stimulus that needed to be remembered. Neurons characterized by sustained activity were also identified in the visual cortex, in the auditory cortex and in the sensorimotor cortex of animals that maintain a particular piece of sensory information in the temporary memory during an exercise that involves visual, auditory and tactile stimuli, respectively. Cf. J. Fuster, "Network memory," *Trends in Neurosciences* 20 (1997): 451–459. It is believed that in each of these cortical areas the sustained neuronal activity signals the participation of the area within a wider network Squire, Kandel, *Memory: from mind to molecules.*

25. Kirwan, Bayley and Squire—C.B. Kirwan et al., "Detailed recollection of remote autobiographical memory after damage to the medial temporal lobe" *Proc Natl Acad Sci U S A.* 105(7) (2008): 2676–2680—have resorted to sensitive tests based on meticulous surveys to recall 50 or more recall details for each memory. An individual's autobiographical recollection proved to be deficient when the memories were about the recent past, while fully intact when they regarded the distant past.

26. It is not known at all to what extent non-human complex organisms have the capacity for episodic memory. Moreover, it has been difficult to conceive of an experiment to solve this problem.

27. This model was developed for the first time by Damasio in 1989 and subsequently incorporated into cognitive theories. See: A. R. Damasio, "Time-locked Multiregional Retroactivation. A Systems-level Proposal for the Neural Substrates of Recall and Recognition," *Cognition* 33: 25–62; W.K. Simmons and L.W. Barsalou, "The Similarity-in-Topography Principle. Reconciling Theories of Conceptual Deficits," *Cognitive Neuropsychology* 20 (2003): 451–86; L. W. Barsalou, "Grounded Cognition," *Annual Review of Psychology* 59 (2008): 617–45.

28. The model takes into account the neuropsychological results of the past twenty years, and postulates that cellular groups at the highest levels of processing hierarchies do not retain explicit representations of the maps of objects and events. They maintain instead the *know-how,* i.e. the *guidelines,* to proceed—if necessary—to the final reconstruction of explicit representations. More specifically, according to Damasio, the guidelines would act on many lower level sensory cortices originally involved in perception: they would do so by means of divergent connections from their site, directed at the lower level sensory cortices. Ultimately, the *locus* where the mnemonic recordings would actually be reproduced would not be very different from that of the original perception. Cf. A. Damasio, *Self Comes to Mind: Constructing the Conscious Brain* (New York: Pantheon, 2010).

29. Damasio defines the auto-biographic self in terms of biographical knowledge relating to both the past and to an anticipation of the future. This is self-conscious human subjectivity (Damasio, *Constructing the Conscious Brain,* 13–14 and 27–28). We will return to this topic later.

30. The genetically modified mice belong to two main categories, respectively known as "knock-out" and "transgenic." In knock-out mice, the gene in question was eliminated from all the cells of the body and remains absent for the entire life of the animal. As a result, the common knock-out genes sometimes lack flexibility and precision: the experimenter does not have the ability to suppress the activity of a gene only in certain cells or only in special moments of the life of the animal. In transgenic mice, on the other hand, a gene is added to the genome, the transgene, by injecting DNA into an egg cell. The transgene can match the *wild-type* (natural) version of the gene in question, in which case the gene product is over expressed, or it can be a mutated version of the gene, designed to enhance or suppress the normal functioning of the same. The transgene also contains a particular promoter element, i.e., a sequence of DNA that controls when (in time) and where (in the body or brain) the gene will be expressed.

31. Our understanding of the nature and function of the genes has given rise, in these last few years, to molecular genetics, a discipline that is now the basis of most biological disciplines. In this context, long-term memory is a topic of vital interest to scholars because it touches on the foundations of the central issues of modern life sciences, allowing us to connect in a profound way the cognitive psychology of a mental process (memory) with molecular biology (protein encoding). Genes are DNA sequences characterized by two important properties, which provide them with a dual purpose. First, they can replicate themselves, acting as a mould, or they can serve as a depository for genetic information, which can be transmitted from one generation to another. Secondly, genes encode the information necessary to produce the proteins that serve as the basis for all aspects of life, including mental processes. Cf. L.R. Squire, "Memory systems of the brain: a brief history and current perspective," *Neurobiol. Learn. Mem.* 82 (3) (2004): 171–177; Id., "Neuroscience. Rapid consolidation," *Science* 316 (5821) (2007): 57–58. The human brain contains about 10^{11} neurons, divided into 1,000 or more cell types. These types can be distinguished by their shape and their specific synaptic connections, that is, they can be distinguished on the basis of certain characteristics determined both by the particular combination of genes expressed by each cell type and by the combination of genes expressed in the respective target cells with which each cell type interacts. The fate of a particular nerve cell, i.e., the type of function it will perform in the brain, is determined by the genes expressed. This decision is made in the early stages of animal development. During ontogeny in a given cell, a particular picture of gene activation and repression occurs, which is typically maintained throughout the life of the cell in question—J. Monod, J. Changeux, and F. Jacob, "Allosteric Proteins and Cellular Control System," *Journal of Molecular Biology* 6 (1963): 306–329. The mechanisms by which genes are turned on and off are important to understanding how the long-term memory is turned on and off. In *Aplysia,* for example, serotonin must somehow regulate gene expression in the sensory neurons of the retraction circuit of the gill in order to induce the formation of new synaptic connections. As we will see later, serotonin performs this particular task, since it activates special regulatory protein molecules that are able to turn certain genes on and off. The way in which genes are turned on and off is a fascinating and important area of research. One fifth of *all* genes of the human genome encode proteins that regulate transcription by activating or inhibiting it. These regulatory transcription proteins coordinate, in turn, the expression of other genes. The discovery that genes can be regulated and the identification of the mechanism behind this adjustment (which is due to Monod's discovery of the Lac operon system) constitutes one of the most important chapters of modern biology—Cf. F. Jacob, J. Monod, "On the Regulation of Gene Activity," *Cold Spring Harbor Symposium on Quantitative Biology* 26 (1961a): 193–211;

Id., "Genetic Regulatory Mechanisms in the Synthesis of Proteins," *Journal of Molecular Biology* 3 (1961b): 318–356. Each gene can be divided into two main regions: an encoding region and a control region or "target" region. The DNA of the "encoding" region can be transcribed into messenger RNA, to be then translated into protein. The fact that a given encoding region is read (transcribed) depends on a number of regulatory proteins able to bind to the control region. The "control" region is generally situated "upstream," i.e., just before the start of the encoding region, and is further divided into two subregions: the "promoter region" and the "regulatory region." The regulatory region, in turn, is divided into some small portions, called DNA "response elements." Each of these response elements recognizes and binds specific "regulatory proteins," called "transcription factors." The latter are of two types: activators, which promote transcription and repressors, which inhibit transcription. These transcription regulators are essential for long-term memory. Alongside the regulatory region, the promoter region binds proteins continuously, determing the steady-state level of transcription in the absence of stimulation. "The various response elements typically bind regulatory proteins only intermittently, as activators and repressors arrive to activate (induce) or repress (shut off) the gene and then depart once they are no longer needed"—Cf. Squire and Kandel, *Memory: from mind to molecules;* Di Bernardo, *Per una rivisitazione della dottrina monodiana;* Id., "Natural selection and self-organization." Here, second messenger systems (each messenger RNa carries information relevant to the production of a specific protein) have the task of signalling different transcription regulators when to bind to certain elements of the response. Therefore, the transcription of a gene and the number of times it is repeated at any given time depends on the transcription regulators that bind to different elements of the region's regulatory response (cf. Kandel et al., *Principles of neural sciences*). The induction of gene expression by the serotonin, which will lead to long-term memory, thus requires the activation of specific transcription factors that can bind to particular response elements of the control region of the genes involved in long-term memory. Therefore, Kandel's idea that the conversion of short-term memory into long-term memory requires the activation of special genes has provided a link between the emerging field of molecular biology of memory storage and the biology of gene regulation, a research field that is already fairly well advanced. Cf. Squire and Kandel, *Memory: from mind to molecules.*

32. This late-phase can be activated by cAMP, one of the molecules of the second messenger system that sends a signal to the nucleus to start gene activation. In a manner similar to what happens in long-term facilitation in *Aplysia,* in the hippocampus of mice, late LTP induces some initial stages during which new proteins are synthesized. Regardless of whether the L-LTP is induced by tetanic stimulation or by the administration of cAMP, its

induction stops when, immediately after tetanic stimulation or during the administration of cAMP, gene transcription is inhibited. The late phase of LTP therefore requires the transcription of certain genes during a critical period that immediately follows the tetanic stimulation, perhaps because during that period particular genes must be expressed. Cf. C.H. Bailey et al., "The persistence of long-term memory: A molecular approach to self-sustaining changes in learning-induced synaptic growth," *Neuron* 44 (2004): 49–57.

33. E. and M. Moser have recently discovered a two-dimensional metric map in the medial entorhinal cortex representing the spatial change of the animal in the environment. An essential component of the medial entorhinal cortex map relates to the presence of nerve cells that send action potentials to multiple locations. The Mosers have termed these nerve cells "grid cells." Grid cells are active in every environment and their intrinsic framework of sending pulses is conserved from one environment to another. This suggests that these cells could be part of a universal mechanism, independent of spatial landmarks, for encoding within the brain the animal's position in space. Grid cells send projections to the hippocampus and furnish the main cortical input for place cells. By combining inputs from different grid cells with different spatial arrangements and orientations, the hippocampal position neurons can generate fields of activity limited to a single location. Unlike the grid cells, the activity of the place cells is highly context-specific, suggesting that positional input coming from the grid cells are integrated with spatial input from other sources to create altogether very different and experience-specific representations. Cf. Squire and Kandel, *Memory: from mind to molecules.*

34. In the course of this research, Kentros and Agnihotri have observed an interesting fact: just as occurs in explicit memory, one key aspect of the stabilization of PKA and of the phase of memory related to the synthesis of new proteins is that of attention. When the mouse does not pay attention to the space in which it moves, the map is formed but is already unstable after few hours. If the mouse is forced to pay attention to its surroundings, the map remains stable for days. Cf. Kandel, "The Molecular Biology of Memory Storage"; Id., *Psychiatry, Psychoanalysis, and the New Biology of Mind* (Washington: American Psychiatric Publishing, 2005).

35. Research carried out by McGaugh and by Dudai have largely extended these results. These scholars have seen that both emotional memory, involving the amygdale, and a type of memory that allows an animal to avoid poisoned food, called 'bait shyness,' and which involves the gustatory area of the cerebral cortex, require a CREB-mediated switch to form long-term memories. Cf. J.M. McGaugh, "Memory: A century of consolidation," *Science* 287 (5451) (2000): 248–251; Y. Dudai, "The neurobiology of consolidations, or, how stable is the engram?" *Ann. Rev. Psychol.* 55 (2004): 51–86).

36. With the term "natural processes" I do not mean to refer to the so-called *methodological naturalism,* typical of empirical research, and much less of the *ontological naturalism* of neo-Darwinian origin, which creates a vision of the world by accepting as true the equating of the totality of experience in becoming with the totality of being (according to this perspective, there would be no trace in humans of any qualitative difference that could justify its special position in relation to other living beings) but rather a new anthropological paradigm that sees in the naturalization of cognitive processes not the threat of materialism, but the opportunity to elevate the biological to a meta-level—Cf. D.J. Siegel, *The Developing Mind* (New York: Guilford Press, 1999); J. Searle, *Mind. A Brief Introduction* (Oxford: Oxford University Press, 2004); G. Edelman, *Wider than the Sky: The Phenomenal Gift of Consciousness* (New Haven: Yale University Press, 2004); Id., *Second Nature: Brain Science and Human Knowledge* (New Haven: Yale University Press, 2006); M. Di Bernardo, "Verso una fondazione naturalistica delle pre-condizioni dell'etica"—where phenomena such as life and consciousness are seen as the result of complex and stratified dialectical processes between three elements in constant mutual interaction, namely, matter, energy and information. Cf. Id., *I sentieri evolutivi della complessità biologica nell'opera di S. A. Kauffman* (Milano: Mimesis, 2011. For an introduction to the philosophical concept of "nature" see: E. Agazzi and N. Vassallo, *Introduzione al naturalismo filosofico contemporaneo* (Milano: Franco Angeli, 1998); M. De Caro and D. Macarthur, eds. *Naturalism and Normativity* (New York: Columbia University Press, 2010); G. Zanet, *Le radici del naturalismo.* W.V. Quine tra eredità empirista e pragmatismo (Macerata: Quodlibet, 2007); S. Semplici, "Il disincanto e la stranezza fino a un certo punto" in *Natura in etica,* eds. F. Botturi and R. Mordacci (Milano: Vita e Pensiero, 2009a), 3–24; Id.,"Il vissuto della mente e la sfida della neuroetica," *Idee* 70 (2009b): 153–67; Grion, L. *Persi nel labirinto. Etica e antropologia alla prova del naturalismo* (Milano: Mimesis, 2012).

Notes to Chapter 3

1. The concept of intentionality was originally developed by Thomas Aquinas and was reintroduced in contemporary philosophy by the philosopher and psychologist Franz Brentano in his book *Psychology from an Empirical Standpoint.* By the intentionality of consciousness or of the mind, he meant the idea that consciousness is always directed towards an object, which always has some content, thus going beyond itself. Brentano defined intentionality as the main feature of *psychic (or mental) phenomena,* through which they may be distinguished from *physical phenomena.* Every mental phenomenon, every psychological act, in fact, has a content, it is

directed to something (the intentional object). Every belief, desire, etc., has an object: that which is believed, that which is desired. Through the works of Husserl, the idea of intentionality entered contemporary research, in both continental and analytic philosophy. In artificial intelligence and cognitive science, intentionality is a controversial issue, regarded as something that a machine could never really have from a structural point of view. Among the supporters of this thesis is Searle, who with his famous Chinese room thought experiment tried to demonstrate the logical impossibility of a machine ever approaching the functioning of the human mind. We will better examine the concept of intentionality, crucial for this work, in the following paragraphs.

2. For Brentano the intentional in-existence exclusively characterises psychic phenomena. No physical phenomenon manifests anything like it. Therefore, we can define psychic phenomena as "those phenomena which contain an object intentionally within themselves" Cf. F. Brentano, *Psychologie vom empirischen Standpunkt* (Hamburg: Felix Meiner Verlag, 1874–1911).

3. Husserl defines the "mental states" endowed with intentionality as intentional *Erlebnisse* or simply *acts* completely avoiding the term "psychic phenomenon" Cf. E. Husserl, *Logische Untersuchungen. Erster Teil: Prolegomena zur reinen Logik* (Halle: Max Niemeyer, 1900); Id., *Logische Untersuchungen. Zweiter Teil: Untersuchungen zur Phänomenologie und Theorie der Erkenntnis* (Halle: Ursula Panzer, 1901).

4. Searle believes that what invalidates traditional approaches, both the materialistic and the dualistic, is the assumption of the "same set of categories inherited from history to describe mental phenomena, consciousness in particular, and, with them, a certain set of assumptions about how consciousness and other mental phenomena relate with each other and with the rest of the world" (Searle, *Mind*, 3). The categories he refers to are the physical and the mental, and the erroneous assumptions underlying these approaches consist of making a clear distinction between physical and mental health, viewing them as mutually exclusive. This way of approaching the problem goes back to Descartes, who said the world is made up of two substances, *res cogitans* and *res extensa*, which differ greatly on an ontological level. The essence of the first is consciousness: it is directly knowable, indestructible and indivisible; the essence of the latter is extension: it is indirectly knowable, divisible and corruptible. The two substances are therefore irreducible and can exist independently of each other. This, however, does not exclude their interaction, as occurs in man, composed of body and soul; in him these two substances interact via the pineal gland. This solution, however, was unable to satisfactorily explain the interaction between the two substances. By laying out the problem in this way, Descartes bequeathed to posterity an important problem, one of the essential issues of the current debate on the nature of the mind and mental states: the problem of the mind-body relationship.

The difficulties incurred by the Cartesian dualism are the same as those of a weaker form of dualism, called "property dualism." This theory holds that there are not two different substances, but two kinds of properties: physical and mental; but this does not facilitate the task of explaining how they act on each other. Searle proposes, against dualism, "an alternative metaphysical picture": we live in a single world, to describe which it is preferable to abandon the categories of physical and mental, because many of its aspects are not covered by them: just think, for example, of money, or the points scored in a football game, or interest rates. Cf. Id., *The Mystery of Consciousness* (New York: The New York Review of Books, 1997).

5. In general, "reductionism" is the term used to describe the perspective that considers the whole to be the sum of its parts; it is often contrasted with the term "holism," which refers to the concept of the whole as an emergent entity, which cannot be reduced to the sum of its parts. For our purposes we can limit ourselves to considering two types of reductionism: one we refer to as *methodological,* and another that we will call *ontological. Methodological reductionism* consists of studying an object by breaking it down ideally into its parts, considered basic, and deducing the properties of the whole from the properties of its elements. This manner of proceeding has yielded great results in scientific research, and can be used successfully, for example, in many fields of physics, but not in all, as evidenced by the discovery of complex dynamic systems, characterized by non-linearity. When speaking instead of *ontological* reductionism, we are referring not only to a methodology of scientific research, but also to a conception of a metaphysical nature, according to which the whole is just the sum of its fundamental parts, so that, ultimately, all the properties of any object in the universe (including human consciousness) would be due to the properties of its constitutive elementary particles; thus we cannot speak of emergent qualities, qualities, that is, that cannot be deduced from the mere sum of the parts. In this perspective, all the sciences, from chemistry to psychology and sociology, would be merely corollaries of elementary particle physics. What we want to emphasize here is that this is a position that cannot be proven solely from within the realm of scientific argument, and therefore it can be sustained or rejected only in relation to one's own particular philosophical system of reference. Cf. J.C. Polkinghorne, "Riduzionismo," in *Dizionario interdisciplinare di scienza e fede,* eds. G. Tanzella-Nitti, A. Strumia (Roma: Urbaniana University Press, 2002), 1231–1236.

6. Searle calls his solution to the mind-body problem *biological naturalism,* i.e., a naturalistic conception which emphasizes the organic nature of mental states, while at the same time avoiding both materialism and dualism. It is a naturalistic solution to the mind, in two senses: first, because mental phenomena are part of nature, and second, because the explanatory apparatus

used to provide a causal explanation of these phenomena is deemed necessary to explain nature in general. Biological naturalism is based on the following four theses: a) mental states, characterized by a first-person ontology, "are real phenomena of the real world": they cannot be eliminated or reduced to brain states, because such a reduction would neglect the first-person ontology; b) everything that is part of our mental life is caused by processes occurring in the brain; c) all mental phenomena are simply features of the brain (and possibly of the central nervous system) and d) as real phenomena of the real world, mental states have "causal efficacy." Cf. Searle, *The Mystery of Consciousness;* Id., *Mind, Language, and society: philosophy in the real world* (New York: Basic Books, 1999); Id., *Rationality in Action* (Cambridge: The MIT Press, 2001); Id., *Mind.* Yet how can the mind, caused by what happens in the brain, be at the same time a feature of what causes it? In effect, Searle explains, this question arises from "misunderstanding causation": when we think of two events joined by a causal relationship, we think of two "discrete" events, separate and distinct from each other, one of which is the cause, the other the effect. In our case, however, he explains, we need a more "sophisticated" understanding of causation. Looking at physics, Searle calls into question the distinction between the microscopic and macroscopic level of a system: consider water, for example. At the microscopic level we find molecules, atoms and subatomic particles; at the macroscopic level, instead, we observe that water is liquid: this is called a surface or global property. A surface property, also called an *emergent property,* is "[. . .] one that is causally explained by the behaviour of the elements of the system; but it is not a property of any individual elements and it cannot be explained simply as a summation of the properties of those elements" (Id., *The Mystery of Consciousness,* 18). Searle efficaciously explains how the surface property is both caused by the behaviour of trace elements, and at the same time created in the system constituted by those trace elements. There is a relationship of cause and effect, but at the same time the surface characteristics are characteristics of the highest level of the same system whose behaviour at the micro level causes those characteristics cf. Id., *Minds, Brains and science* (Cambridge: Harvard University Press, 1984). The same considerations should be made for the mind and the brain: it is in this sense that brain processes cause mental states, which in turn are realized in the system constituted by neurons. Furthermore, Searle adds, just as we can refer to a system of particles, but not to the individual particles, as being liquid or solid, so we can refer to a brain as conscious, but not to a neuron as being so. Searle thus elaborates a theory of mind that goes in the direction of a "non-reductionist naturalization": a 'naturalization' because, as mentioned, the mental states exist and are part of nature just like digestion and photosynthesis; 'non-reductionist' because these states are not identified, as was the case in some forms of materialism, with brain states, although they are caused by them. It should be added that the form of reductionism Searle condemns is ontological reductionism, which consists in showing that objects of a certain type, in this case mental states, are nothing more than objects of another type, that is, brain states; he does not critique, but rather makes his own, what is referred to as causal reduction whereby we can say that "phenomena of type A are *causally reducible* to phenomena of type B, if and only if the behavior of A is entirely causally explained by the behavior of B, and A's behavior has no causal powers beyond those of B" (Id., *Mind,* 119): the liquidity of water can be reduced causally to the behaviour of molecules and mental states are causally, and not ontologically, reducible to brain states. One could argue, Searle notes, that as in the case of water, where we can reduce liquidity to the movement and structure of the molecules composing it, in the same way one could reduce the mind to brain states. This reduction, however, cannot be performed because one cannot distinguish in these cases between appearance and reality: "[. . .] if it consciously seems to me that I am conscious, then I am conscious" (Id., *Mind,* 122); I can be deceived about the contents of my states, but not about their consciousness. This is another way, Searle writes, of saying that the mental possesses a first-person ontology and therefore cannot be ontologically reduced to what possesses a third-person ontology. If we wish to ontologically reduce mental states to configurations of neurons, we will lose the essential properties of these states. When you have a thought, what is really happening is that brain activity is taking place. Brain activity causes bodily movements through physiological processes. Therefore, since mental states are brain characteristics, they have two levels of description: a higher level (what we referred to above as the macro level of a system) described in mental terms, and a lower level (micro level) described in physiological terms; a single action can be described on both levels. For further discussion of the concept of biological naturalism see: M. Velmans and S. Schneider. eds. *The Blackwell companion to consciousness* (Malden: Wiley-Blackwell, 2008).

7. For further discussion of this topic see: G. Cosmacini, *La medicina non è una scienza. Breve storia delle sue scienze di base* (Milano: Raffaello Cortina, 2008).

8. It seems useful, in this respect, to propose here, in agreement with Penna and Pessa, a distinction between two different types of connectionism, which we will refer to respectively as strong and weak, analogous to the attributes used for the two forms of artificial intelligence. Strong connectionism, exemplified by the work of researchers such as Hinton and Dyer—G. Hinton, ed. *Connectionist symbol processing* (Cambridge: MIT Press, 1991); M. Dyer, "Distributed symbol formation and processing in connectionist networks," *Journal of Experimental and Theoretical Artificial Intelligence* 2 (1990): 215–239)—is an emergentist theory: it argues that in a complex system of processing

units interacting with each other and with the outside world, collective processes may arise, which come to constitute "emergent" entities with a life of their own, independent of that of the individual units. These new emergent entities can be identified with thought, with semantics, etc. One can therefore assert, in principle, according to strong connectionism, that a neural network might even think. Weak connectionism, however, considers neural networks merely a more convenient way to create more efficient artificial processing devices. The question of whether the network can think is never asked, since such a problem goes beyond the level at which one operates whenever such models are needed. It is clear that Searle's argument goes against strong connectionism and that its validity is based on the supposed equivalence between connectionist models and programs. Cf. M.P. Penna and E. Pessa, *Introduzione alla psicologia connessionista* (Roma: Di Renzo, 1998); E. Pessa and M.P. Penna, *Manuale di scienza cognitiva. Intelligenza artificiale classica e psicologia cognitiva* (Roma-Bari: Laterza, 2004).

9. We consider as a form of materialistic monism, albeit of a refined type, the idea that consciousness is a mental process that emerges from the *quantitative complexity* of interactions between the many components of the system. This is Kandel's view and in part also that of Damasio: not distinguishing between surface and depth information, they reduce intentional causation to efficient causality, thereby inverting the roles of the effect (molecular syntax) and the cause (meaning). For them, in addition, the concept of information cannot be separated from that of the material support; they also reduce quality to quantity and reduce the temporality that brings about new features to linear space. Cf. E.R. Kandel, *In Search of Memory: The Emergence of a New Science of Mind* (New York: W.W. Norton & Company, 2006), 10–12; Damasio, *Self Comes to Mind,* 40–41.

10. For further discussion, see Di Bernardo, "Natural selection and self-organization"; Id., I sentieri evolutivi della complessità biologica; Id., "Memoria, coscienza e plasticità sinaptica. Esplorazioni epistemologiche," Información Filosófica 9 (19) (2012): 90–125.

11. For further discussion of this topic, we refer the reader to: Id., "Verso una fondazione naturalistica delle pre-condizioni dell'etica."

12. Autocatalysis is a catalytic process in which the catalyst is one of the same products or reaction intermediates capable of acting on the slow stage of the chemical reaction. Common examples of autocatalysis are tin plague (an allotropic modification), the depletion of the ozone layer, hemoglobin's oxygen bonding and the reaction between permanganate and oxalic acid (Mn^{2+} is the autocatalyst). For further discussion see: I. Prigogine and I. Stengers, *La Nouvelle alliance. Métamorphose de la science* (Paris: Gallimard, 1979); S.A. Kauffman, *The Origins of Order: Self-Organization and Selection in Evolution* (New York: Oxford University Press, 1993).

13. For a discussion of the concept of "second nature" revisited in a neurobiological and philosophical key, we refer the reader to Edelman, *Wider than the Sky;* Id., *Second Nature;* Semplici, "Il disincanto e la stranezza fino a un certo punto"; Id.,"Il vissuto della mente e la sfida della neuroetica."

14. In *Reinventing the Sacred,* however, Kauffman recognizes that binary logic and the NK models are, in fact, idealizations designed, however, to understand some of the real mechanisms of memory and consciousness-S.A. Kauffman, *Reinventing the Sacred. A New View of Science, Reason and Religion* (New York: Basic Books, 2008), 105.

15. The denial of free will, according to Freeman, follows from considering the brain inserted within a linear causal chain. Since linear causality is the product of the intentional mechanism by which the brain builds knowledge and since it is out of place to attribute it to complex material systems, contrasting free will with determinism creates an illusory problem. There is no intentional action independent of its historical context or totally constrained by genetic and environmental determinants. The deterministic nature-culture dualism (a kind of Aristotelian law of the excluded middle) fails to take into account the capacity of intentional beings to create and pursue their own personal goals within the social context. Even with the same genetic endowment (as in the case of identical twins) each individual chooses a different and unique direction to develop their own potential. Attributing choices to random noise is to admit that no known cause can be assigned it. In other words, in agreement with Freeman, free will and universal determinism are the contradictory conclusions to which linear causality leads, and the only way out is to deny freedom by assuming randomness, or to deny causality except as an action in a social context by an intentional being. Cf. W.J. Freeman, "Role of chaotic dynamics in neural plasticity," *Progress in Brain Research* 102 (1994): 319–333; Id., *How Brains Make up Their Minds* (New York: Columbia University Press, 2000a); Id., "Indirect biological measures of consciousness from field studies of brains as dynamical systems," *Neural Networks* 20 (2007): 1021–1031.

16. In recent decades, biology has become the subject of increasing analysis by philosophers, especially because of the delicacy of the issue at stake, that is, life, and of the different perspectives through which it can be understood today. If a philosophy of science applied to quantum mechanics is able to interest itself in issues such as causality, indeterminacy or the nature of time, when the subject of discussion is life, its origin and its evolution, then philosophical reflections surely cannot fail to investigate, directly or indirectly, even deeper questions, sometimes capable of reaching the realm of the existential and the theological. This is demonstrated by the broad debate on the philosophical implications of biological evolution and the most recent and equally extensive debate that today accompanies the re-evaluation

by contemporary biology of the concept of "information." Evidence of this are the numerous works carried out almost in parallel by scholars such as Kauffman, Fox Keller, Maynard Smith, Davies, Gregersen, Atlan, Carsetti, Floridi, Vedral, Avery, Talmy and which in recent years through a vast scientific production, are bearing fruit by placing before the attention of the international community a number of interesting insights. Cf. Kauffman, *Reinventing the sacred;* Fox Keller, *Making Sense of Life: Explaining Biological Development with Models, Metaphors, and Machines* (Cambridge: Harvard University Press, 2003); Id., *The Mirage of a Space between Nature and Nurture* (Durham: Duke University Press, 2010); J. Maynard Smith, "The concept of information in biology" *Philosophy of Science* 67 (2000): 177–194; P. Davies and N. Gregersen. eds. *Information and the nature of reality. From physics to metaphysics* (Cambridge: Cambridge University Press, 2010); H. Atlan, *Le vivant post-génomique ou Qu'est-ce que l'auto-organisation?* (Paris: Odile Jacob, 2011); A. Carsetti, "The embodied meaning and the unfolding of the mind's eyes," in *New essays in logic and philosophy of science,* ed. D. D'Agostino and G. Giorello, SILFS (London: College Publications, 2010b), 539–547; Id., *Epistemic complexity and knowledge construction. Morphogenesis, symbolic dynamics and beyond* (Berlin: Springer, 2013); L. Floridi, *The Philosophy of Information* (Oxford: Oxford University Press, 2011); V. Vedral, *Decoding Reality: The Universe as Quantum Information* (New York: Oxford University Press, 2010); J. Avery, *Information theory and evolution* (Singapore: World Scientific, 2003); L. Talmy, *Toward a cognitive semantics* (Cambridge: MIT Press, 2000).

17. The relationship between memory and neuroscience, as we have seen, implies the need to consider a serious philosophical problem (related to the issue of reductionism): how should we describe a system in which there are different levels of activity connected by both bottom-up and top-down relations? If we don't face this question, we can do nothing but reproduce implicitly the old Cartesian mind-body dualism, with all the absurdities that result. Unfortunately, the problem is far from being resolved in a definitive manner. The solution proposed by physicists, with tools such as statistical mechanics, the theory of phase transitions and emergence, complexity theory, classical or quantum mechanics, is still very limited and inadequate for the biological, psychological and social world. The concept of a fixed point, on which Carsetti—"Randomness, information and meaningful complexity: some remarks about the emergence of biological structures," *La Nuova Critica* 36 (2000b): 47–109; "The emergence of meaning at the co-evolutionary level: An epistemological approach," *Int. Jour. of Applied Mathematics and Computation.* 219 (2012a): 14–23; *Epistemic complexity and knowledge construction*—has been working for many years, allows us to take several important steps towards a solution (allowing us to expand beyond

the classical version of complexity theory), but requires considerable further technical efforts, in the mathematical sense of the term. In other words, in current scientific thought, we are waiting for a new Newton capable of making the physical and mathematical sciences take a jump a similar, but much more far-reaching, than what the great English scholar had done with physics and mathematics four centuries ago at the dawn of modernity. In particular, we are waiting for an adequate theory of information for physical systems that do not fall within the paradigm of systems of classical mechanics—including statistical mechanics—such as stable nonlinear dynamical systems out of equilibrium (chaotic systems). A theory of information, thus, that is adequate (true) for all biological and cognitive systems.

18. On this level, according to the perspective outlined in these pages, in offering us the possibility of understanding the nature of human processes of categorial intuition, only the phenomenological method will allow us to avoid both the dangers of Idealism, with its risk of an inevitable drift towards a new metaphysics, and Neopositivism's instant rejection of all possible forms of metaphysics.

19. Here the term 'consciousness' [*coscienza*] is understood in the English sense of consciousness, which indicates self-reflexivity. In Italian and in the human sciences often the term *coscienza* instead often refers to "moral conscience." In this sense, talking about natural processes applied to memory and consciousness, means identifying "natural processes" with "human processes" typical of the human species understood as a species in nature. Finally, as regards moral conscience, according to this perspective, we can infer that what are natural are surely its pre-conditions that reside in intentionality, a fundamental characteristic of the *bios*. The great mystery for neurobiology is thus not so much the meta-reflexive human act present in some vertebrates (albeit in minimal forms), but the existence in man of a free will (which is experienced at every moment) that cannot be formalised and is absolutely incompressible since it is pure creativity. Cf. Di Bernardo, "Verso una fondazione naturalistica delle pre-condizioni dell'etica"; Id., "Memoria, coscienza e plasticità sinaptica."

Notes to chapter 4

1. The discovery of so called "mirror neurons," that is neurons whose activation corresponds to observation of an action by another living being as well as the carrying out of the action by the individual has opened up new perspectives. Specifically if the same circuit is activated when an action takes place, independently of whether the action is carried out by the body which contains the circuit it would appear that there is an equivalence between activity intended as concrete action and the interpretation of the activity

itself. Some of the neurons of this group seem to be activated on the basis of the purpose of the action and not the way that this is carried out. In fact, the imitation of the gesture of grasping in the absence of the object to be taken does not activate the neuron: one possible interpretation is that the how of the action is not important, it is the "what" for activation. If indeed a certain group of neurons is activated not just when a certain kind of movement is carried out but only when this movement takes on a clear goal (grasping a cracker to bring it to the mouth activates mirror neurons, carrying out the same gesture without a cracker does not), the temptation to interpret this phenomena in terms of "knowledge equals the assumption of one's own point of view as the origin of meaning" is strong. The activation of the "mirror" group of neurons (confirmed experimentally) seem to indicate that the action itself goes beyond a purely physical analysis of the observed gesture. Indeed when faced with what could be described as univocal stimuli in terms of physical description (cleaning a window with a circular gesture or waving the hand in greeting), but that produce different opinions and judgments, there are three interpretative possibilities: a different sensation, a different perception or a different interpretation of the signal. The first case is within the context of the purely structural aspect of the nervous system involving practically only the most peripheral part and is almost totally definable with objective scientific methods. Already in the second case aspects that are not possible to render objective assume an important role. We should think, then, what is the role played by past experience and culture in the definition of the stimulus. The significance that the gesture assumes, indeed depends on the environmental context but also on conventions: think of the way Italians and Americans count on their fingers (one starts counting one with the thumb, the other with the index finger). Even the circuit mechanism is not completely defined with regard to aspects relating to pure perception of stimuli. Furthermore there is the problem of the interpretation of the gesture and the stimulus, a consequence of the fact that this is, by definition, subjective and therefore falls outside the field of the objective sciences Cf. C. Cerri, "Attività neurale ed espressione personale, nesso di causalità o causalità organizzata?" in *Intenzionalità ed empatia. Fenomenologia, psicologia, neuroscienze,* M. Armezzani et al (Roma: Edizioni OCD, 2008).

2. The presence of others is connected in Husserl's reflections to giving oneself the objective thing and bodily presence: I take the world not only as my world but as a horizon inhabited by other presences "analogous" to mine. The exercise of *epoché* shows the presence to be structurally ambiguous, as a "lived duality" between psychic and corporeal being. When I put everything that I have learned about my conscience and my mind to one side "the paradox of human subjectivity which is both subject for the world and object in the world" is revealed. This experience of "lived duality" signifies "foreign

belonging" and "immanent transcendence." The structural non-coincidence with myself that I find in living in my body, in my temporal and possible determinations, in my not completely explicit presence, this other than "my own" has, as Husserl says, priority with respect to the constitution of any external objectivity and enables me to perceive the other as an "alien analogue." Cf. E. Husserl, (1921–28) *Zur Phänomenologie der Intersubjektivität. Texte aus dem Nachlass* (Netherlands: Martinus Nijhoff, 1973); Id. (1931) *Cartesianische Meditationen und Pariser Vorträge* (Dordrecht: Kluwer, 1950); Id. *Ideen II: Phänomenologische Untersuchungen zur Konstitution* (Dordrecht: Kluwer, 1952a); Id. *Ideen III: Die Phänomenologie und die Fundamente der Wissenschaften* (Dordrecht: Kluwer, 1952b).

3. "From this point of view, if we can talk about perceptive intelligence as a transversal function with respect to the various levels of consciousness, in the same way we can hypothesize that a hierarchical vision of memory (which starts in the sensorial and motor sphere and goes as far as configuring areas of association in which declarative and somatic memory are carried out) is reinterpretable in the light of a modular consideration of memory, though in its vertical aspect, according to which memories of different qualities are interconnected both in the first phases of their formation and in the continuum of their development, and there are not postulated sequential, logical and chronological criteria that separate horizontally (in the sense of successive steps) the activation of the various types of memory " C. Sabatano, *Come si forma la memoria. Ipotesi sperimentali di ricerca bioeducativa* (Roma: Carocci, 2004), 13.

4. Here the concept of nature is widened to consider the physical and psychic as references of the spiritual and the person as a dialectic synthesis of the complex relationships that exist between three different existential levels: body, mind and spirit (see Husserl, *Ideen II).* It is at this level that it is possible to think, in agreement with Hegel, of the existence of a second nature. This concept has been studied in neuroscience by C. McGinn, *Knowledge and Reality: Selected Essays* (New York: Oxford University, 1999); Edelman, *Second Nature;* Semplici, "Il vissuto della mente e la sfida della neuroetica."

5. Some of the more prominent studies done recently in this area are those by Amari—"Information Geometry on Hierarchy of Probability Distributions," *Ieee Transactions on Information Theory* 47 (5) (2001): 1701–11-, Freeman—*Neurodynamics: An Exploration of Mesoscopic Brain Dynamics* (London: Springer-Verlag, 2000b); "A pseudo-equilibrium thermodynamic model of information processing in nonlinear brain dynamics," *Neural Networks* 21 (2008): 257–265—D. Harter and R. Kozma,—"Aperiodic Dynamics and the Self- Organization of Cognitive Maps in Autonomous Agents," *Int. J. Intelligent Systems* 21 (9) (2006): 955–972—, Vitiello—Coherent states, fractals and brain waves. *New Mathematics and Natural Computing* 5 (2009b): 245–264. They

involve what we might now call a third AI, aimed not at simulating the human mind, but rather at understanding its systemic and integrated nature through toy models (with new components such as memristors, artificial synapses, etc.) and abundant doses of differential geometry (collective behaviours). The basic idea is very simple. The collective neural behaviors can be described in geometrodynamic terms. The modification of these geometries thus serves as a measure of information and its changes. There are three types of neural systems: a) without input (absolutely unrealistic); b) input-output (very toylike, but they involve an environment and an elementary goal, such as "I'm hungry, I fill my plate with pasta") and finally c) "intentional behaviors." Following Freeman's lead (and the Turing test), we do not claim to say what they consist of, rather, but limit ourselves to describing what could be defined as their neurogeometric correlative elements. It is interesting to note that for there to be intentional behaviors, there must necessarily be an environment and therefore, "noise"; the minimum cost function (the brain is a physical device) shows in this case more complex behaviors than in the first two cases, and shows an oscillating pattern around a task (plurality of choices) that can be expressed as a percolating around a phase trajectory. Cf. I. Licata, Beyond Turing: Hypercomputation and Quantum Morphogenesis. *Asia Pacific Mathematics Newsletter.* 2 (2012): 20–24; I. Licata, G. Resconi, "Geometry for a Brain. Optimal Control in a Network of Adaptive Memristors," *Adv. Studies Theor. Phys.* 7 (10) (2013): 479–513. For further discussion of the relationship between visual perception and neurogeometry see: A. Carsetti, "The emergence of meaning at the co-evolutionary level: An epistemological approach," *Int. Jour. of Applied Mathematics and Computation.* 219 (2012a): 14–23; J. Petitot, "The neurogeometry of pinwheels as a sub-Riemannian contact structure," *Journal of Physiology* 97 (2003): 265–309; Id., *Neurogéometrie de la vision* (Paris: Les Editions de l'Ecole Polytechnique); Id., "Neurogeometry of neural functional architectures," *Chaos, Solitons & Fractals* 50 (2008): 75–92; G. Longo, "Theorems as constructive visions," in *Proof and Proving in Mathematics Education. New ICMI Study,* vol. 15, eds. G. Hannade, M. Villiers. (Berlin: Springer, 2012): 51–66.

6. Consider for example the work on the topic of realism by A. Eddington, *The Nature of the Physical World* (Ann Arbor: University of Michigan Press, 1958); K.R. Popper, *Objective Knowledge: An Evolutionary Approach* (Oxford: Clarendon Press, 1972); H. Maturana and F. Varela, *Autopoiesis and Cognition: The Realization of the Living* (Dordrecht: Reidel, 1980); H. Putnam, *The Marry Faces of Realism* (La Salle: Open Court Press, 1987).

7. For an introduction to functional realism see: F. Wuketits, "Self-organization, Constructivism, and Reality," *La Nuova Critica* 17–18 (1991): 21–36; Id., "Self-organization, complexity and the emergence of human consciousness," *La Nuova Critica* 19–20 (1992): 89–109; Id., "Functional

realism," in *Functional models of cognition,* ed. A. Carsetti (Dordrecht: Kluwer Academic Publisher, 2000), 27–38; J. Götschl and W. Leinfellner, "Erwin Schrödinger's world view. The role of physics and biology in his philosophical system." in *What is Controlling Life? 50 years after Erwin Schrödinger's What is Life?* In *Modern Trends in BioThermoKinetics,* eds E. Gnaiger et al. vol. 3. (Innsbruck: University Press, 1994); A. Carsetti, "Processi epigenetici e strutture riflessive nel sistema nervoso centrale," *La Nuova Critica* 69–70 (1984a): 79–117; Id., "Evoluzione naturale e teoria algoritmica della complessità," *La Nuova Critica* 71–72(1984b): 42–82; Id., "Linguaggi, procedure del riferimento e realtà," in *Contesti e validità del discorso scientifico,* ed. L. Cuccurullo and E. Mariani (Rome, 2005a), 262–279.

Works Cited

Works cited in the preface:

Cariani, P. 2011. The semiotics of cybernetic percept-action systems. *International Journal of Signs and Semiotic Systems* 1(1): 1–17.

Chemero, A. 2009. *Radical Embodied Cognitive Science*. MIT Press.

Deco, G., E.T. Rolls, and R. Romo. 2009. Stochastic dynamics as a principle of brain function. *Progress in Neurobiology* 88 :1–16.

Doya, K, S. Ishii, and A. Puget. 2011. *Bayesian Brain: Probabilistic Approaches to Neural Coding*. MIT Press.

Gallagher, S., and D. Zahavi. 2008. *The Phenomenological Mind. An Introduction to Philosophy of Mind and Cognitive Science*. Routledge.

Gibson, J. J. 1986. *The Ecological Approach to Visual Perception*. Lawrence Erlbaum.

Haikonen, P.O. 2007. *Robot Brains: Circuits and Systems for Conscious Machines*. Wiley-Interscience.

Huys, R. et al. 2008. Distinct Timing Mechanisms Produce Discrete and Continuous Movements. *PLoS Comput Biol* 4(4): e1000061. doi:10.1371/journal.pcbi.1000061.

Kauffman, S. 2009. *Physics and Five Problems in the Philosophy of Mind*. ArXiv: 0907.2494v1 [Physics.hist-ph].

Licata, I. 2008. Logical Openness in Cognitive Models. *Epistemologia* 31: 177–192.

———, and A. Sakaji. (eds.). 2008. *Physics of Emergence and Organization*. World Scientific.

Maturana, H, and F. Varela. 1992. *Tree of Knowledge*. Shambhala.

Resconi, G. 2013. *Geometry of Knowledge for Intelligent Systems*. Springer.

Rozenberg, G., T. Bäck, and J.N. Kok. eds. 2012. *Handbook of Natural Computing*. Springer.

Scott, A. 1995. *Stairway to the Mind. The Controversial New Science of Consciousness*. Springer.

VanRullen, R., and C. Koch. 2003. Is perception discrete or continuous? *Trends Cogn. Sci.* 7 (5): 207–213.

Works cited in the text:

Abel, T. et al. 1997. Genetic demonstration of a role PKA in the late phase of LTP and in hippocampus-based long-term memory. *Cell,* 88: 615–626.

Agazzi, E., 1999. *Paideia verità educazione,* Brescia: La Scuola.

Ainsworth, M.D.S. et al. 1978. *Patterns of Attachment: A Psychological Study of the Strange Situation.* Erlbaum: Hillsdale.

Albright T.D., T. M. Jessell, E.R. Kandel, and M.I. Posner. 2000. Neural science: a century of progress and the mysteries that remain. *Cell.* 100: S1–S55.

Ales Bello, A. 1999. Empatia e dialogo: un'analisi fenomenologica. In *Dialogo, Silenzio, Empatia,* ed. A. Dentone, and M. Bracco, Foggia: Bastogi.

Ammaniti, M. 1989. (ed.). *La nascita del sé.* Roma-Bari: Laterza.

Andrews, K. et al. 1996. Misdiagnosis of the vegetative state: retrospective study in a rehabilitation unit. *BMJ* 313: 13–16.

Aquinas, T. 1265–1274. *Summa Theologica.* Notre Dame (IN): Ave Maria Press (1981).

Armezzani, M. 2008. Gli psicologi e l'empatia. Atteggiamenti e stili di ricerca di fronte alla sfida della fenomenologia e delle neuroscienze. In *Intenzionalità ed empatia. Fenomenologia, psicologia, neuroscienze,* M. Armezzani et al. Roma: OCD, 63–91.

Astolfi L. et al. 2009. *The* track of brain activity during the observation of TV commercials with the high-resolution EEG technology, *Comput Intell Neurosci.*: 652078.

Atlan, H. 1985. Complessità, disordine e auto-creazione del significato. In *La sfida della complessità,* eds. G. Bocchi, and M. Ceruti. Milano: Mondadori (2007), 134–154.

———. 1987. Self creation of meaning. *Phys. Scr.* 36: 563–76.

———. 1998. Intentional self-organization. Emergence and reduction. Towards a physical theory of intentionality. *Thesis Eleven* 52: 5–34.

———. 2000. Self-organizing networks: weak, strong and intentional, the role of their underdetermination, in *Functional models of cognition. Self-organizing dynamics and semantic structures in cognitive systems,* ed. A. Carsetti, Dordrecht: Kluwer, 127–142.

———. 2011. *Le vivant post-génomique ou Qu'est-ce que l'auto-organisation?* Paris: Odile Jacob.

Atlan, H. and Y. Louzoun. 2007. Emergence of intentional procedures in self-organizing neural networks. *La Nuova Critica* 49–50: 67–81.

Baccarini, E. 2002. *La soggettività dialogica*, Roma: Aracne.

———. 2003. *La persona e i suoi volti*, Roma: Anicia.

Baddeley, A.D., and G. Hitch. 1974. *Working memory*. In *The psychology of learning and motivation: Advances in research and theory*, ed. G.H. Bower. New York: Academic Press, 47–89.

———. 2000. The episodic buffer: a new component of working memory? *Trends in Cognitive Science* 4: 417–423.

———. 2004. *Your Memory: A User's Guide*. New York: Firefly Books.

Bailey, C.H., and M. Chen. 1988. Long-term memory in Aplysia modulates the total number of varicosities of single identified sensory neurons. *Proceeding of the National Academy of Sciences of the USA* 85: 2373–2377.

———. 1989. Time course of structural changes at identified sensory neuron synapses during long-term sensitization in Aplysia. *Journal of Neuroscience* 9: 1774–1780.

Barrow-Green, J. 1997. *Poincaré and the Three Body Problem*. Providence (RI): Amer. Math. Soc.

Bartlett, F. 1951. *The mind at work and play*. London: Allen and Unwin.

———. 1958. *Thinking*. New York: Basic Books.

Basti, G. 2011. Intelligence and reference. Formal ontology of the natural computation. STOQ-Science. Roma: Lateran University Press.

Bekinschtein, T.A. et al. 2011. Functional imaging reveals movement preparatory activity in the vegetative state. *frontiers in Human Neuroscience* 5: 1–13.

Bellingreri, A. 2005. *Per una pedagogia dell'empatia*. Milano: Vita e Pensiero.

———. 2006. *Il superficiale il profondo. Saggi di antropologia pedagogica*, Milano: Vita e Pensiero.

Benedersky, M., and M. Lewis. 1994. Environmental risk, biological risk, and developmental outcome. *Developmental Psycology* 30: 484–494.

Bergson, H. 1907. *L'Evolution créatrice*. 86th ed. Paris: Les Presses universitaires de France (1959).

Bernat, J.L. 2002. Questions remaining about the minimally conscious state. *Neurology* 58: 337–338.

Bisiach, E., and C. Luzzati. 1978. Unilateral neglect of representational space. *Cortex* 14: 129–133.

Blasone, M., and G. Vitiello. 2011. *Quantum Field Theory and its Macroscopic Manifestations*. London: Imperial College Press.

Bliss, T., and T. Lomo. 1973. Long-lasting potentiation of synaptic transmission in the dentate area of the anaesthetized rabbit following stimulation of the perforant path. *J Physiol*. 232(2): 331–56.

Bliss, T., G. Collingridge, and L. Morris. (eds). 2004. *Long-term Potentiation: Enhancing Neuroscience for 30 years*. New York: Oxford University Press.

Bocchi, G., and M. Ceruti. (ed.) 2007. *La sfida della complessità*, Milano: Mondadori.

Boella, L. 2008. *Neuroetica. La morale prima della morale*. Milano: Raffaello Cortina.

Bolshakov, V.Y. et al. 1997. Recruitment of new sites of synaptic transmission during the cAMP-dependent late phase of LTP at CA3-CA1 synapses in the hippocampus. *Neuron* 19: 635–651.

Boly, M. et al. 2011. Preserved feedforward but impaired top-down processes in the vegetative state. *Science*. 332 (6031): 858–62.

Bourtchouladze, R.A. et al. 1994. Deficient long-term memory in mice with a targeted mutation of the cAMP responsive element binding protein. *Cell* 79: 59–68.

Bowlby, J. 1979. *The Making and Breaking of Affectional Bonds*. London: Tavistock.

Bruner, J. S. 1983. *Child's Talk: Learning to use Language*. Oxford: Oxford University Press.

———. 1986. *Actual Minds, Possible Worlds*. London: Harvard University Press.

———. 1993. *Acts of Meaning. Four Lectures on Mind and Culture*. Cambridge: Harvard University Press.

———. 1994. The Remembered Self, in *The Remembering Self: Construction and Accuracy in the Self Narrative*, ed. U. Neisser, and R. Fivush. Cambridge: Cambridge University Press, 41–54.

———. 1996. *The culture of education*. Cambridge (MA): Harvard

University Press.

Buffalo, E.A. et al. 2010. A backward progression of attentional effects in the ventral stream. *Proc Natl Acad Sci U S A.* 107(1): 361–5.

Buzzoni, M. 2008. *Thought Experiment in the Natural Sciences. A Transcendental-Operational Conception.* Würzburg: Königshausen +Neumann.

Byrne, J.H., V.F. Castellucci, and E.R. Kandel. 1974. Receptive fields and response properties of mechanoreceptor neurons innervating skin and mantle shelf of Aplysia. *Journal of Neurophysiology* 37: 1041–1064.

Byrne, J.H. et al. 1978. Stimulus-response relations and stability of mechanoreceptor and motor neurons mediating defensive gill-withdrawal reflex in Aplysia. *Journal of Neurophysiology* 41: 402–417.

Callari Galli, M. et al. 2005. *Formare alla complessità.* Roma: Carocci Editore.

Calvet, J., and J. Coll. 1959. Meningitis of sinusoid origin with the form of coma vigil. *Rev Otoneuroophtalmol.* 31: 443–445.

Capecchi, M. 1990. Gene targeting. How efficient can you get? *Nature.* 348(6297): 109.

Carnap R, and Y. Bar-Hillel. 1952. *An outline of a theory of semantic information.* Technical Report N. 247. Cambridge (MA): MIT Press.

Carsetti, A. 1984a. Processi epigenetici e strutture riflessive nel sistema nervoso centrale. *La Nuova Critica* 69–70: 79–117.

———. 1984b. Evoluzione naturale e teoria algoritmica della complessità. *La Nuova Critica* 71–72: 42–82.

———. 1987. Teoria algoritmica della informazione e sistemi biologici. *La Nuova Critica* 3–4: 37–66.

———. 1988. Probability, Randomness and Information, in *Probability in the Sciences,* ed. E. Agazzi, Dordrecht, 165–75.

———. 1989. Teoria della complessità e modelli della conoscenza. *La Nuova Critica* 9–10: 61–103.

———. 1991. Complessità e significato. In *Realismo, Semantica Formale e Teoria della Complessità,* Bologna, 1–20.

———. 1999. Mental constructions and non-standard semantics. *La Nuova Critica* 33–34:101–126.

———. 2000a. Linguistic structures, cognitive functions and algebraic semantics. In *Functional models of cognition. Self-organizing dynamics and semantic structures in cognitive systems*, ed. Id., Dordrecht: Kluwer, 253–286.

———. 2000b. Randomness, information and meaningful complexity: some remarks about the emergence of biological structures. *La Nuova Critica* 36: 47–109.

———. 2004. The embodied meaning: self-organisation and symbolic dynamics in visual cognition. In *Seeing, thinking and knowing. Meaning and self-Organisation in Visual Cognition and Thought*, ed. Id., Dordrecht: Kluwer, 307–330.

———. 2005a. Linguaggi, procedure del riferimento e realtà. In *Contesti e validità del discorso scientifico*, ed. L. Cuccurullo, and E. Mariani, Roma, 262–279.

———. 2005b. Entropia, morfogenesi autonoma e sistemi cognitivi. *La Nuova critica* 45–46: 59–105.

———. 2006.. Functional realism, non-standard semantics and the genesis of the minds'eyes. *La Nuova Critica* 47–48: 171–197.

———. 2007. Natural language, categorisation processes and the self-organising cognitive code. *La Nuova Critica* 49–50:181–215.

———. 2008. Significato, verità ed in comprimibilità. La costruzione "meaning-oriented" di spazi concettuali d'ordine superiore e la modulazione primaria, a livello coevolutivo, del codice semantico proprio della mente umana, PRIN.

———. 2009a. Knowledge construction, non-standard semantics and the genesis of the mind's eyes. In *Causality, meaningful complexity and embodied cognition*, ed. Id., Berlin: Springer, 283–300.

———. 2009b. Embodiment processes and intentional complexity. *La Nuova Critica* 53–54:103–122.

———. 2010a. Complexity, self-organisation and natural evolution. In *Handbook of Evolution*. vol. 3, ed. F. M. Wuketits, New York.

———. 2012a. The emergence of meaning at the co-evolutionary level: An epistemological approach. *Int. Jour. of Applied Mathematics and Computation*. 219: 14–23.

———. 2012b. Eigenforms, natural computing and morphogenesis. Turing Centenary Conference.

———. 2013. *Epistemic complexity and knowledge construction. Morphogenesis, symbolic dynamics and beyond*. Berlin: Springer.

Castellucci, V.F. et al. 1970. Neuronal mechanisms of habituation and dishabituation of the gill-withdrawal reflex in Aplysia. *Science* 167: 1745–1748.

———. et al. 1980. Intracellular injection of the catalytic subunit of cyclic AMP–dependent protein kinase simulates facilitation of transmitter release underlying behavioral sensitization in Aplysia. *Proc Natl Acad Sci* 77: 7492–7496.

Chaitin, G. 1974. Information-theoretic computational complexity. *IEEE Trans. Inf. Th.* IT–20: 10–15.

———. 1987. *Algorithmic information theory*. Cambridge: Cambridge University Press.

———. 1990. *Information, Randomness, and Incompleteness*. Singapore: World Scientific.

Churchland, P.S. 2002. *Brain-Wise: Studies in Neurophilosophy*. Cambridge: The MIT Press.

———. 2013. *Touching A Nerve: The Self As Brain*. W. W. Norton & Company.

Churchland, P.S., and T.J. Sejnowski. 1992. *The Computational Brain*. Cambridge: The MIT Press.

Cincotti, F. et al. 2003. The use of EEG modifications due to motor imagery for brain-computer interfaces. IEEE Trans Neural Syst Rehabil Eng. 11(2): 131–3.

Cincotti F. et al. 2007. Vibrotactile feedback for brain-computer interface operation. *Comput Intell Neurosci*: 48937.

Cincotti F. et al. 2008. Non-invasive brain-computer interface system: towards its application as assistive technology. *Brain Res Bull*. 75 (6): 796–803.

Ciompi, L. 1991. Affects as Central Organising and Integrating Factors: A New Psychosocial/Biological Model of the Psyche. *British Journal of Psychiatry* 159: 97–105.

Coleman, M. *et al*. 2009. Towards the routine use of brain imaging to aid the clinical diagnosis of disorders of consciousness. *Brain* 132(Pt 9): 2541–2552.

Collins, A.M., and M.R. Quillian. 1969. Retrieval time from semantic memory. *Journal of Verbal Learning and Verbal Behavior* 8 : 240–47.

Collins, A.M., and E.F. Loftus. 1975. A spreading-activation theory of semantic processing. *Psychological Review*. 82 (6): 407–428.

Craik, F.I.M., and E. Tulving. 1975. Depth of processing and the retention of words in episodic memory. *Journal of Experimental Psychology*. 104: 268–294.

Cruse D., and A.M. Owen. 2010. Consciousness revealed: new insights into the vegetative and minimally conscious states. *Curr Opin Neurol*. 23 (6): 656–60.

Damasio, A. R. 1989. Time-locked Multiregional Retroactivation. A Systems-level Proposal for the Neural Substrates of Recall and Recognition. *Cognition* 33: 25–62.

———. 1994. *Descartes' Error: Emotion, Reason, and the Human Brain*. New York: Putnam.

———. 1999. *The Feeling of What Happens: Body and Emotion in the Making of Consciousness*, New York: Harcourt.

———. 2003. *Looking for Spinoza: Joy, Sorrow, and the Feeling Brain*. New York: Harcourt.

———. 2007. Neuroscience and Ethics. Intersections. *American Journal of Bioethics* 7(1): 3–7.

———. 2010. *Self Comes to Mind: Constructing the Conscious Brain*. New York: Pantheon.

Darwin, C.R. 1902. *On the Origin of Species by Means of Natural Selection or The Preservation of Favoured Races in the Struggle for Life*. H. Frowde. London: Oxford University Press.

———. 1958. *The Autobiography of Charles Darwin 1809–1882. With the*

Original Omissions Restored. Edited and with Appendix and Notes by his Granddaughter Nora Barlow. London: Collins.

Dehane, S. et al. 2006. Conscious, preconscious, and subliminal processing: a testable taxonomy. *Trends Cogn Sci* 10: 204–211.

Del Re, G. 2000. *The Cosmic Dance*. Randor: Templeton Found Press.

Dennet, D. C. 1995. *Darwin's Dangerous Idea: Evolution and the Meanings of Life*. New York: Simon & Schuster.

Di, H. et al. 2008. Neuroimaging activation studies in the vegetative state: predictors of recovery? *Clin. Med.* 8: 502–507.

Di Bernardo, M. 2007. *Per una rivisitazione della dottrina monodiana della morfogenesi autonoma alla luce dei nuovi scenari aperti dalla post-genomica*. Roma: Aracne.

———. 2010. Natural selection and self-organization in complex adaptive systems. *Rivista di Biologia / Biology Forum* 103 (1): 75– 96.

———. 2011, *I sentieri evolutivi della complessità biologica nell'opera di S. A. Kauffman*. Milano: Mimesis.

———. 2012. Memoria, coscienza e plasticità sinaptica. Esplorazioni epistemologiche. *Información Filosófica* 9 (19): 90–125

Di Francesco, M. 1998. *L'io e i suoi sé. Identità personale e scienza della mente*. Milano: Raffaello Cortina.

Ebbinghaus, H. 1885. *Memory: A contribution to experimental psychology*. New York: Dover.

Edelman, G. 1987. *Neural Darwinism: The Theory of Neuronal Group Selection* New York: Basic Books.

———. 1990. *The Remembered Present: A Biological Theory of Consciousness*. New York: Basic Books.

———. 2004. *Wider than the Sky: The Phenomenal Gift of Consciousness*. New Haven: Yale University Press.

———. 2006. *Second Nature: Brain Science and Human Knowledge*. New Haven: Yale University Press.

Edelman, G., Tononi, G. 2000. *A Universe of Consciousness: How Matter Becomes Imagination*. New York: Basic Books.

Engert, F., and T. Bonhoeffer. 1999. Dendritic spine changes associated with hippocampal long-term synaptic plasticity. *Nature* 399: 66–70.

Fasolo, B., G.H. McClelland, and K.A. Lange. 2005. The effect of site design and interattribute correlations on interactive web-based decisions. In *Online Consumer Psychology: Understanding and influencing behavior in the virtual world*, eds. CP Haugtvedt, K. Machleit, and R. Yalch, New Jersey: Lawrence Erlbaum Associates.

Fernández-Espejo, D. et al. 2010. *Diffusion weighted imaging distinguishes the vegetative state from the minimally conscious state. NeuroImage* 54: 103–112.

Fodor, J.A. 1975. The language of thought. Cambridge (MA): Harvard University Press.

———. 1983. *Modularity of Mind: An Essay on Faculty Psychology*. Cambridge (MA): MIT Press.

Foulkes, S. H. 1975. *Group Analytic Psychotherapy*. London: Gordon and Breach.

Fox Keller, E. 2000. *The Century of the Gene*. Cambridge (MA) Harvard University Press.

———. 2010. *The Mirage of a Space between Nature and Nurture*. Durham: Duke University Press.

Frankl, V. 1972. *10* Thesen über die Person, in *Der Wille zum Sinn. Ausgewählte Vorträge über Logotherapie,* Bern-Stuttgart-Wien: Verlag Hans Huber, 108–118.

Frankland, P.V. et al. 2004. The involvement of the anterior cingulated cortex in remote contextual fear memory. *Science* 304: 881–883.

Frauenfelder E.1983, *La prospettiva educativa tra biologia e cultura,* Napoli: Liguori.

———. 1986. *Educazione e processi apprenditivi: elementi per una pedagogia dell'apprendimento.* Napoli: Tecnodid.

———. 2001. *Pedagogia e biologia. Una possibile alleanza*. Napoli: Liguori Editore.

Frauenfelder, E. and F. Santoianni. 1997. *Nuove frontiere della ricerca pedagogica tra bioscienze e cibernetica.* Napoli: Edizioni Scientifiche Italiane.

———. (eds.). 2002. *Le scienze bioeducative. Prospettive di ricerca,* Napoli: Liguori.

———. 2003a. *Percorsi dell'apprendimento, percorsi dell'insegnamento.* Roma: Armando.

———. 2003b. Mind, Learning and Knowledge in Educational Contexts. Research Perspectives in Bioeducational Sciences. Cambridge Scholars Press.

Frauenfelder E., F. Santoianni, and M. Striano. 2004. *Introduzione alle scienze bioeducative,* Roma-Bari: Laterza.

Frazier, W.T. et al. 1967. Morphological and functional properties of identified neurons in the abdominal ganglion of Aplysia californica. *Journal of Neurophysiology* 30: 1288–1351.

Freeman, W. J. 1994. Role of chaotic dynamics in neural plasticity. *Progress in Brain Research* 102: 319–333.

———. 1995. *Societies of Brains*. Mahwah (NJ): Lawrence Erlbaum Associates.

———. 1997. Nonlinear neurodynamics of intentionality, *Journal of Mind and Behavior* 18 (2–3): 291–304.

———. 2000a. *How Brains Make up Their Minds.* New York: Columbia University Press.

———.2000b. *Neurodynamics: An Exploration of Mesoscopic Brain Dy-*

namics. London: Springer-Verlag.

———. 2004. *How* and why brains create MEANING-T from sensory information. *International Journal of Bifurcation & Chaos* 14: 513–530.

———. 2006. Origin, structure, and role of background EEG activity. Part 4. Neural frame simulation. *Clin. Neurophysiol* 117: 572–589.

———. 2007, Indirect biological measures of consciousness from field studies of brains as dynamical systems. *Neural Networks* 20: 1021–1031.

———. 2008. A pseudo-equilibrium thermodynamic model of information processing in nonlinear brain dynamics. *Neural Networks* 21: 257–265.

Freeman, W. J., and G. Vitiello. 2006. Nonlinear brain dynamics as macroscopic manifestation of underlying many-body field dynamics. *Physics of Life Reviews* 3: 93–118.

———. 2008. Dissipation and spontaneous symmetry breaking in brain dynamics. *J. Phys. A: Math. Theor* 41: 304042.

———. 2009. Dissipative neurodynamics in perception Forms cortical patterns that are stabilized by vortices. *J. Phys. Conf. Ser,* 174 (012011): 1–24.

Freeman, W. J., and R. Quian Quiroga. 2013. *Imaging Brain Function with EEG: Advanced Temporal and Spatial Analysis of Electroencephalographic Signals.* Berlin: Springer.

Frege, G. 1892. Über Sinn und Bedeutung. *Ztschr. f. Philos. u. philos. Kritik,* 100: 25–50.

Frey, U. et al. 1993. Effects of cAMP simulate a late stage of LTP in hippocampal CA1 neurons. *Science* 260: 1661–1664.

Fuster, J. 1997. Network memory. *Trends in Neurosciences* 20: 451–459.

Gabora, L. et al. 2013. A Quantum Model of Exaptation: Incorporating Potentiality into Evolutionary Theory. *Progress in Biophysics & Molecular Biology,* 113(1): 108-116.

Gallese, V. et al. 1996. Action recognition in the premotor cortex. *Brain,* 119: 593–609.

Gallese, V. 2006. Corpo vivo, simulazione incarnata e intersoggettività. Una prospettiva neuro fenomenologica. In *Neurofenomenologia,* ed. M. Cappuccio. Milano: Mondadori.

———. 2007. Dai neuroni specchio alla consonanza intenzionale.

Meccanismi neurofisiologici dell'intersoggettività. *Rivista di Psicoanalisi* 53 (1): 197–208.

———. 2008. Mirror neurons and the social nature of language: the neural exploitation hypothesis. *Soc Neurosci* 3 (3–4): 317–33.

———. 2009. Motor abstraction: a neuroscientific account of how action goals and intentions are mapped and understood. *Psychol Res*. 73(4): 486–98.

Gardner, H. 1991. *The Unschooled Mind*. New York: Basic Books.

Gazzaniga, M.S. 2006. Facts, Fictions and the Future of Neuroethics. In *Neuroethics. Defining the Issues in Theory, Practice and Policy*, ed. J. Illes. Oxford-New York: Oxford University Press.

Gervilla, E. 2000. Un modelo axiológico de educación integral. *Revista Española de Pedagogía* 58: 39–57.

Giacino, J.T. et al. 2002. The minimally conscious state: Definition and diagnostic criteria. *Neurology*. 58 (3): 349–353.

Giannone F., and G. Lo Verso. 1996. *Il Self e la polis. Il sociale e il mondo interno*. Milano: Franco Angeli.

Gödel, K. 1972. Kurt Gödel: Collected Works, I, II, III (eds. S. Feferman et al. 1986, 1990, 1995). Oxford: Oxford University Press.

Goldsmith, H. H., K.A. Buss, and K.S. Lemery. 1997. Toddler and childhood temperament: Expanded content, stronger genetic evidence, new evidence for the importance of environment. Developmental Psychology 33, 891–905.

Gosseries, O. et al. 2011. Disorders of consciousness: what's in a name? NeuroReabilitation, 28: 3–14.

Grant, S.G. et al. 1992. Impaired long-term potentiation, spatial learning, and hippocampal development in fyn mutant mice. Science. 258(5090): 1903–10.

Grasselli, G. and P. Strata. 2013. Structural plasticity of climbing fibers and the growth-associated protein GAP-43. *Frontiers in neural circuits*, 7: 25.

Grion, L. 2012. *Persi nel labirinto. Etica e antropologia alla prova del naturalismo*. Milano: Mimesis.

Grossberg, S. 1988. Neural Networks and Natural Intelligence. Cambridge (MA): MIT Press.

———. 2004. Neural Models of Seeing and Thinking, in Seeing, Thinking and Knowing. Meaning and Self-Organisation in Visual

Cognition and Thought, ed. A. Carsetti. Dordrecht: Kluwer: 29–54.

Hagen, M.C. et al. 2002. Tactile Motion Activates in the Human Middle Temporal/V5 (MT/V5) Complex. *European Journal of Neuroscience*, 16: 957–64.

Hagmann, P. et al. 2008. Mapping the Structural Core of Human Cerebral Cortex. *PloS Biology* 6(7): e159.

Haken, H. 2006. *Information and Self-Organization: A Macroscopic Approach to Complex Systems*, Berlin: Springer.

Halbwachs, M. 1992. *On Collective Memory*. Chicago: University of Chicago Press.

Hall, W.A. et al. 2001. Minimally invasive procedures. Interventional MR image-guided neurobiopsy. *Neuroimaging Clin N Am*. 11(4): 705–13.

Harvey, C.D., and K. Svoboda. 2007. Locally dynamic synaptic learning rules in pyramidal neuron dendrites. *Nature* 450(7173): 1195–200.

Hawkins, R.D., V.F. Castellucci, and E.K. Kandel. 1981. Interneurons involved in mediation and modulation of the gill-withdrawal reflex in Aplysia, II: Identified neurons produce hetero-synaptic facilitation contributing to behavioral sensitization. *Journal of Neurophysiology* 45: 315–326.

Hebb, D.O. 1949. *The Organization of Behavior: A Neuropsychological Theory*. New York: Wiley.

Hintikka, J. 1970. *Surface information and depth information*. In *Information and inference*, eds. J. Hintikka, and P. Suppes. Dordrecht: Reidel, 298–330.

Hintzman, D.L. 1986. "Schema abstraction" in a multiple trace memory model. *Psychological Review* 93: 411–28.

Hopfield, J.J. 1982. Neural networks and physical systems with emergent collective computational abilities. *Proceedings of the National Academy of Sciences of USA*, 79: 2554–2558.

Husserl, E. 1908. *Vorlesungen über Bedeutungslehre.* Netherlands: Martinus Nijhoff (1987).

———. 1931. *Cartesianische Meditationen und Pariser Vorträge*. Dordrecht: Kluwer (1950).

———. 1939. *Erfahrung und Urteil. Untersuchungen zur Genealogie der*

Logik. Hamburg: Felix Meiner Verlag GmbH (1999).

———. 1952a. *Ideen II: Phänomenologische Untersuchungen zur Konstitution*. Dordrecht: Kluwer.

———. 1952b. *Ideen III: Die Phänomenologie und die Fundamente der Wissenschaften*. Dordrecht: Kluwer.

Iacoboni, M. 2008. *Mirroring people. The Science of Empathy and How We Connect with Others*. New York: Picador.

Jablonka, E., and M.J. Lamb. 2005. *Evolution in Four Dimensions. Genetic, Epigenetic, Behavioral and Symbolic Variation in the History of Life*. Cambridge (MA): MIT Press.

Jacob F., 1977. Evolution and Tinkering. *Science* 196: 1161–1166.

———. 1982. *The possible and the actual*. New York: Pantheon.

———. 1983. Molecular tinkering in evolution. In *Evolution from melecules to men*, ed. D.S. Rondall. Cambridge: Cambridge University Press.

James, W. 1879. Are we automata? *Mind*, 4: 1–21.

———. 1890. *The Principles of Psychology*. New York: Henry Holt.

Jaynes, E. T. 1965. Gibbs vs Boltzmann Entropies. *Am. J. Phys.*, 33: 391.

———. 2000. *The Origin of Consciousness in the Breakdown of the Bicameral Mind*. New York: Mariner Books.

Kandel, E.R. 1975. Perspectives in the neurophysiological study of behavior and its abnormalities. In *New Psychiatric Frontiers: American Handbook of Psychiatry*, 2nd ed. eds. D. A. Hamburg, and H.K.H. Brodie. New York: Basic Books.

———. 1976. *Cellular basis of behavior: an introduction to behavioral biology*, San Francisco: W. H. Freeman.

———. 1978. A cell-biological approach to learning. Grass Lecture Monograph 1, Society for Neuroscience.

———. 1979a. Psychotherapy and the single synapse: the impact of psychiatric thought on neurobiological research. *New England Journal of Medicine* 310: 1028–1037.

———. 1979b. Small systems of neurons. *Scientific American* 241: 66–76.

———. 1983a. From metapsychology to molecular biology: explorations into the nature of anxiety. *Am. J. Psychiatry* 140 (10): 1277–93.

———. 1983b. Neurobiology and molecular biology: the second encounter. *Cold Spring Harb Symp Quant Biol.* 48 (2): 891–908.

———. 1989. Genes, nerve cells, and remembrance of things past. *Journal of Neuropsychiatry and Clinical Neurosciences* 1: 103–125.

———. 1997. Genes, synapses, and long-term memory. *J. Cell. Physiol.* 173 (2): 124–5.

———. 1998. A new intellectual framework for psychiatry. *American Journal of Psychiatry* 155: 103–125.

———. 1999. Biology and the future of psychoanalysis: a new intellectual framework for psychiatry revisited. *Am. J. Psychiatry* 156 (4): 505–24.

———. 2001. The Molecular Biology of Memory Storage: A Dialogue Between Genes and Synapses. *Science* 294 (5544): 1030–1038.

———. 2005. *Psychiatry, Psychoanalysis, and the New Biology of Mind.* Washington, DC: American Psychiatric Publishing, Inc.

———. 2006. *In Search of Memory: The Emergence of a New Science of Mind*. New York: W.W. Norton & Company.

———. 2009. The biology of memory: a forty-year perspective. *J. Neurosci.* 29 (41): 12748–56.

———. 2012. The molecular biology of memory: cAMP, PKA, CREB-1, CREB-2, and CPEB. *Mol. Brain.* 5: 14.

———., and W.A. Spencer. 1961. Electrophysiological properties of an archicortical neuron. *Annals of the New York Academy of Sciences* 94: 570–603.

———. 1968. Cellular neurophysiological approaches in the study of learning. *Physiological Reviews* 48: 65–134.

———. et al. 1976. A common presynaptic locus for the synaptic changes underlying short-term habituation and sensitization of the gill-withdrawal reflex in Aplysia. *Cold Spring Harbor Symposia on Quantitative Biology* 40: 465–482.

———., and L.R. Squire. 2000. Neuroscience: breaking down scientific barriers to the study of brain and mind. *Science* 290 (5494): 1113–20.

———., J.H. Schwartz, and T.M. Jessell. 2000. *Principles of neural sciences*, 4th ed. New York: The McGraw-Hill Companies.

———., and C. Pittenger. 2003. Past and future studies of memory. *Kos.* 211: 38–43.

Kant, I. 1797. *Die Metaphysik der Sitten.* English: *The Metaphysics of Morals*. Cambridge: Cambridge University Press (1991).

Kauffman, S. A. 1993. *The Origins of Order: Self-Organization and Selection in Evolution*. New York: Oxford University Press.

———. 1995. *At Home in the Universe: the Search of the Laws of Self-Organization and Complexity*. New York: Oxford University Press.

———. 2000. *Investigations*. New York: Oxford University Press.

———. 2008. *Reinventing the Sacred. A New View of Science, Reason and Religion*. New York: Basic Books.

Kauffman, S. A. et al. 2008. Critical networks exhibit maximal information diversity in structure-dynamics relationships. *Phys. Rev. Lett.* 100 (5): 058702.

Kentros, C. et al. 1998. Abolition of long-term stability of new hippocampal place cell maps by NMDA receptor blockage. *Science* 280: 2121–2126.

———. et al. 2001. Stabilization of the hippocampal representation of space in mice requires attention. *Abstracts of the Society of Neoscience* 27: 316–315.

Kiefer, M. et al. 2008. The Sound of Concepts. Four Markers for a Link Between Auditory and Conceptual Brain Systems. *Journal of Neuroscience* 28: 12224–30.

Kim, J.H. et al. 2003. Presynaptic activation of silent synapses and growth of new synapses contribute to intermediate and long-term facilitation in Aplysia. *Neuron*. 40 (1): 151–65.

Kolmogorov, A. 1965. Three approaches to the quantitative definition of information. *Problem in Information Transmission* 1: 3–11.

Lakoff, G., and M. Johnson. 1999. *Philosophy In The Flesh: the Embodied Mind and its Challenge to Western Thought*. New York: Basic Books.

Lakoff, G., and R. Nuñez. 2001. *Where Mathematics Comes From: How the Embodied Mind Brings Mathematics into Being*. New York: Basic Books.

Landry, C.D., E.K. Kandel, and P. Rajasethupaty. 2013. New mechanism in memory storage: piRNAs and epigenetics. *Trends Neurosci.* S0166–2236 (13): 00103–3.

Laplace, P.S. 1776. Recherches sur l'intégration des équations différentielles aux différences finies et sur leur usage dans la théorie des hasards. *Mém. Acad. R. Sci.* Paris (Savants Étrangers) 7 (1773). OC 8: 69–197.

Laureys, S. 2004. Functional neuroimaging in the vegetative state.

NeuroRehabilitation. 19 (4): 335–41.

———. 2005. The neural correlate of (un)awareness: lessons from the vegetative state. *Trends Cogn Sci*. 9: 556–559.

———. 2007. Eyes open, brain shut. *Sci Am*. 296 (5): 84–9.

———. et al. 1999. Cerebral metabolism during vegetative state and after recovery to consciousness. *J Neurol Neurosurg Psychiatry* 67: 121–122.

———. et al. 2000. Auditory processing in the vegetative state. *Brain* 123(Pt 8): 1589–1601.

———., and M. Boly. 2007. What is it like to be vegetative or minimally conscious? *Curr Opin Neurol*. 20(6): 609–13.

———. et al. 2010. Consciousness, Unresponsive wakefulness syndrome: a new name for the vegetative state or apallic syndrome», *BMC Med* 8: 68.

———., and N.D. Schiff. 2012. Coma and consciousness: paradigms (re)framed by neuroimaging. *Neuroimage*. 61(2): 478–91.

Le Doux, J. E. 1996. *The Emotional Brain: The Mysterious Under pinnings of Emotional Life*. New York: Simon & Schuster.

———. 2002. *Synaptic Self: how our brains become who we are*, New York: Viking Penguin.

Licata, I. 2008. *La logica aperta della mente*. Torino: Codice Edizioni.

———. 2011. *Complessità. Un'introduzione semplice*. Palermo: Duepunti Edizioni.

Licata, I., and A. Sakaji. 2008. *Physics of Emergence and Organization*, Singapore: World Scientific.

Lo Coco, G., and G. Lo Verso. 2006. *La cura relazionale. Disturbo psichico e guarigione nelle terapie di gruppo*. Milano: Raffaello Cortina Editore.

Loeb C., and G.F. Poggio. 1998. *Le basi cerebrali della mente*. Roma: Universo.

Lo Verso G. 1989. *Clinica della gruppoanalisi e psicologia*. Torino: Bollati Boringhieri.

———. 1994. *Le relazioni soggettuali*. Torino: Bollati Boringhieri.

———., and C. Prestano. 2003. Relational Goods: Costs and Effectiveness. *Group Analysis* 36: 539–547.

Luria, A. 1980. *Higher Cortical Functions in Man*. New York: Basic Books.

Mansuy, I.M. et al. 1998. Restricted and regulated overexpression reveals calcineurin as a key component in the transition from short-term to long-term memory. *Cell* 92: 39–49.

Marciani, M.G. et al. 1996. Effect of lamotrigine on EEG paroxysmal abnormalities and background activity: a computerized analysis. *Br J Clin Pharmacol.* 42 (5): 621–7.

———., and F. Placidi. 2009. Coma, alterazioni della coscienza e sonno. In *Malattie del Sistema Nervoso*, C. Ferrarese et al. Milano: McGraw-Hill Companies, 115–120.

———. 2011. Stato vegetativo e stato di minima coscienza: aspetti clinici, etici e giuridici. Roma: Ateneo Pontificio Regina Apostolorum.

Marshall W.H., C.N. Woolsey, and P. Bard. 1937. Cortical representation of tactile sensibility as indicated by cortical potentials. *Science* 85 (2207): 388–90.

Martin, A. et al. 1998. Synapse-specific transcription dependent long-term facilitation of the sensory to motor neuron connection in Aplysia: A function for local protein synthesis in memory storage. *Cell* 91: 927–938.

Massimini, M. et al. 2012. Cortical mechanisms of loss of consciousness: insight from TMS/EEG studies. *Arch Ital Biol.* 150 (2–3): 44–55.

Maturana, H.R., and F. Varela. 1973, *De maquinas y seres vivos*. Santiago de Chile: Editorial Universitaria.

———. 1980. *Autopoiesis and Cognition: The Realization of the Living*. Dordrecht: Reidel.

———. 1992. *The Tree of Knowledge: the biological toots of human understanding*, Boston: Shambhala.

Maturana, H.R. 1975. The organization of the living: a theory of the living organization. *Int. J. Machine Studies* 7: 3–34.

———. 1978. Biology of language: The epistemology of reality. In *Psychology and biology of language and thought: Essay in honor of Eric Lenneberg*, eds. G. A. Miller and E. Lenneberg. New York: Academic Press, 27–63.

———. 1997. *Objectivity - An argument to force*. Santiago de Chile: Ed Dolmen.

———. 2007. The nature of the laws of nature. *Systems research and behavioral science* 17 (5): 459.

Mayford, M. et al. 1996. Control of memory formation through regulated expression of a CaMKII transgene. *Science* 274: 1678–1683.

McDougall,W. 1924. *Ethics and some modern world problems*. New York: Putnam.

Merleau-Ponty, M. 1942. *La Structure du comportement*. Paris: Presses Universitaires de France.

———. 1945. *Phénoménologie de la perception*. Paris: Gallimard.

———. 1964. *Le Visible et l'invisible, suivi de notes de travail*. Paris: Gallimard.

Merzenich, M.M., and K. Sameshima. 1993. Cortical plasticity and memory. *Curr. Opin. Neurobiol.* 3 (2): 187–96.

Mesulam, M. M. 1998. Review Article:From Sensation to Cognition. *Brain* 121: 1013–1052.

Meyer, D.E. 1970. On the representation and retrieval of stored semantic information. *Cognitive Psychology* 1: 242–249.

Meyer, K., and A. Damasio. 2009. Convergence and Divergence in a Neural Architecture for Recognition and Memory. *Trends in Neurosciences* 32(7): 376–82.

Milner B. 1962. Les troubles de la memoire accompagnant des lesions hippocampiques bilaterales. In *Physiologie de l'hippocampe*, ed. P. Passouant. Paris: Centre National de la Recherche Scientifique, 257–272.

———. 1966. Amnesia following operation on the temporal lobes. In *Amnesia*, eds. C.W.M. Whitty, and O.L. Zangwill. London: Butterworths, 109–133.

———. et al. 1968. Further analysis of the hippocampal amnesic syndrome: 14-year follow-up study of HM. *Neuropsychologia* 6: 215–234.

———., L.R. Squire, and E.K. Kandel. 1998. Cognitive Neuroscience and the Study of Memory. *Neuron*, 20: 445–468.

Miano, F. 2003. *Dimensioni del soggetto*. Roma: AVE.

———. 2009, *Responsabilità*. Napoli: Guida.

Minati, G., *et al.* (eds.). 2008. *Processes of emergence of systems and systemic properties. Towards a general theory of emergence*. Singapore: World Scientific.

Mittelstaedt, P. 1990. The interrelation between Language and Reality in Quantum Physics. *La Nuova Critica* 13–14: 89–109.

Monod, J. 1970. *Le hasard et la necessite: essai sur la philosophie naturelle de la biologie moderne*. English: *Chance and Necessity. An Essay on the National Philosophy of Modern Biology*. Glasgow: Collins Fontana Books (1974).

Montarolo, P.G. et al. 1986. A critical period for macromolecular synthesis in long-term heterosynaptic facilitation in Aplysia. *Science* 234: 1249–1254.

Monti, M.M., S. Laureys, and A.M. Owen. 2010. The vegetative state. *BMJ*. 341: c3765.

Naci, L., and A.M. Owen. 2013. Making Every Word Count for Nonresponsive Patients. *Jama Neurol*.

Nagel, T. 1978. *The Possibility of Altruism*. Princeton (NJ): Princeton University Press.

———. 1991. Conoscenza e realtà oggettiva. In *L'automa spirituale*, eds. G. Giorello, and P. Strata. Roma-Bari: Laterza.

———. 1995. *Other Minds: Critical Essays. 1969–1994*. New York: Oxford University Press.

———. 2012. *Mind and Cosmos: Why the Materialist Neo-Darwinian Conception of Nature is Almost Certainly False*. New York: Oxford University Press.

Napolitani, D. 1987. *Individualità e gruppalità*, Torino: Bollati Boringhieri.

Neisser, U., and I. Hyman. 2000. Memory Observed: Remembering in Natural Contexts. 2nd ed. New York: Worth Publishers.

Nguyen, P.V. et al. 1994. Requirement of a critical period of transcription for induction of a late phase of LTP. *Science* 265: 1104–1107.

Nicolis, G., and I. Prigogine. 1977. *Self Organization in Non-Equilibrium Systems*. New York: J. Wiley and Sons.

Nicolis G., and I. Prigogine. 1989. *Exploring Complexity: an introduction*. New York: Freeman & Co.

Nicoll, R.A., J. A. Kauer, and R.C. Malenka. 1988. The current excitement in long-term potentiation. *Neuron*.1(2): 97–103.

Nietzsche, F. 1881. *Morgenröthe. Gedanken über die moralischen Vorurtheile*. Paderborn: Salzwasser Verlag (2011).

Noirhomme, Q. et al. 2010. Brain connectivity in pathological and pharmacological coma. *frontiers in Systems Neuroscience* 4: 1–6.

O'Keefe, J., and L. Nadel. 1978. *The Hippocampus as Cognitive Map.*

Clarendon: Oxford University Press.

Oliverio Ferraris, A. and A. Oliverio. 2007. *Psicologia. I motivi del comportamento umano*. Bologna: Zanichelli.

Oliverio, A. 2008. *Geografia della mente. Territori cerebrali e comportamenti umani*. Milano: Raffaello Cortina.

———. 2013. *Immaginazione e memoria. Fantasia e realtà nei processi mentali*. Milano: Mondadori.

Omodeo, P. 1984. Che cos'è un organismo vivente? Il contributo della teoria dell'informazione. *La Nuova Critica* 71–72: 31–42.

Owen, A.M. 2008. Disorders of consciousness. *Ann N Y Acad Sci*.1124: 225–38.

———. 2013. Detecting consciousness: a unique role for neuroimaging. *Annu Rev Psychol*. 64: 109–33.

———. et al. 2005. Residual auditory function in persistent vegetative state: a combined PET and fMRI study. *Neuropsychol Rehabil* 15: 290–306.

———. et al. 2006. Detecting awareness in the vegetative state. *Science* 313: 1402.

———. et al. 2007. Functional MRI in disorders of consciousness: advantages and limitations. *Curr Opin Neurol* 20: 632–637.

———., et al. 2009. A new era of coma and consciousness science. *Progress in Brain Research* 177: 399–411.

Panfield, W., and T. Rasmussen. 1952. *The Cerebral Cortex of Man: A Clinical Study of Localization of Function*. New York: Macmillan.

———. 1952. Memory mechanisms. *AMA Arch. Neurol. Psychiatry* 67 (2): 178–98.

———. 1958. Functional localization in temporal and deep sylvian areas. *Res. Publ. Assoc. Res. Ment. Dis.* 36: 210–226.

Pavlov, I. P. 1927. *Conditioned Reflexes: An Investigation of the Physiological Activity of the Cerebral Cortex.* London: Oxford University Press.

Penna, M.P., and E. Pessa. 1998. *Introduzione alla psicologia connessionista*. Roma: Di Renzo.

———. 1996. *Le interfacce uomo-macchina*. Roma: Di Renzo.

Pessa, E. 1992. *Intelligenza Artificiale. Teorie e sistemi*. Torino: Boringhieri.

———. 1993. *Reti neurali e processi cognitivi*. Roma: Di Renzo.

———. 1998. Emergence, Self-Organization, and Quantum Theory. In

First Italian Conference on Systemics, ed G.Minati. Milano: Apogeo, 59–79.

———. (2000) Connectionist Psychology and Synergetics of Cognition. In *Functional Models of Cognition. Self-Organizing Dynamics and Semantic Structures in Cognitive Systems*, ed. A.Carsetti. Dordrecht: Kluwer, 67–90.

———. 2012. On Models of Emergent Metastructures. In On Models of Emergent Metastructures. Methods, Models, Simulations and Approaches Towards a General Theory of Change, eds. G. Minati, M. Abram, E. Pessa. Singapore: World Scientific: 113–132.

Pessa, E., and M.P. Penna. 1994. *La rappresentazione della conoscenza. Introduzione alla Psicologia dei Processi Cognitivi*. Roma: Armando.

———. 2004. *Manuale di scienza cognitiva. Intelligenza artificiale classica e psicologia cognitiva*. Roma-Bari: Laterza.

———., and G. Vitiello. 1999. Quantum dissipation and neural net dynamics. *Bioelectrochemistry and Bioenergetics* 48: 339–342

Petitot, J. 2008. *Neurogéometrie de la vision*. Paris : Les Editions de l'Ecole Polytechnique.

———. 2013. Neurogeometry of neural functional architectures. *Chaos, Solitons & Fractals* 50: 75–92.

Piaget, J. 1971. *Biology and Knowledge*. Chicago: University of Chicago Press.

———. 1973. *Memory and intelligence.* New York: Basic Books.

Pibram, K. H. 1969. *The Four R's of Remembering: Memory Mechanism.* New York: Penguin.

Pinsker, H.M. et al. 1970. Habituation and dishabituation of the gill-withdrawal reflex in Aplysia. *Science* 167: 1740–1742.

———. et al. 1973. Long-term sensitization of a defensive withdrawal reflex in Aplysia. *Science* 182: 1039–1042.

Posner, J.B. et al. 2007. *Plum and Posner's diagnosis of stupor and coma.* Forth Edition. New York: Cambridge University Press.

———. et al. 2009. The neurophysiological bases of emotion: an fMRI study of the affective circumplex using emotion-denoting words. *Hum. Brain Mapp.* 30: 883–895.

Post, R. M., and S.R.B. Weiss. 1997. Emergent properties of neural systems: How focal molecular neurobiological alterations can affect behavior. *Development and Psychopathology* 9: 907–930.

Prigogine, I. 1980. *From Being to Becoming*. San Francisco: W.H. Freeman.

———. 1988. Origin of Complexity, in *Origins: The Darwin College Lectures*, ed. A. C. Fabian. Cambridge: Cambridge University Press: 69–89.

———. 1993. *Les lois du Chaos*. Paris: Flammarion.

———, and I. Stengers. 1979. *La Nouvelle alliance. Métamorphose de la science*. Paris: Gallimard.

———. 1984. *Order Out of Chaos*. New York: Bentham Books.

———. 1988. *Entre le temps et l'éternité*. Paris: Fayard.

Quian Quiroga, R. 2013. Meaning from sensory information. *Physics of Life Reviews* 10: 101–102.

Ramon y Cajal, S. 1894. The Croonian Lecture: La fine structure des centres nerveux. *Proceedings of the Royal Society of London. Series B: Biological Sciences* 55: 444–467.

———. 1906. The structure and connexions of neurons. In *Nobel Lectures: Physiology or Medicine (1901–1921)*. Amsterdam: Elsevier (1967): 220–253.

———. 1911. Histologie du système nerveux de l'homme et des vertébrés, Vols 1 and 2. Paris: A Maloine. Reprinted by Consejo Superior de Investigaciones Cientificas, Inst. Ramón y Cajal, Madrid, 1955.

———. 1937. *1852–1934. Recollections of My Life*. Philadelphia: American Philosophical Society (1989).

Reid, L.H. et al. 1991. Cotransformation and gene targeting in mouse embryonic stem cells. *Mol Cell Biol.* 11(5): 2769–77.

Rispoli, L., and B. Andriello. 1988. *Psicoterapia corporea e analisi del carattere.* Torino: Bollati Boringhieri.

Rizzolatti, G. et al. 1996. Premotor cortex and the recognition of motor actions. *Cogn. Brain Res.* 3: 131–141.

Rizzolatti, G., E. Fogassi, and V. Gallese. 2001. Neurophysiological mechanisms underlying the understanding and imitation of action. *Nature Neuroscience Reviews* 2: 661–670.

———. 2002. Motor and cognitive functions of the ventral premotor cortex. *Current opinions in neurobiology* 12: 149–154.

———. 2006. Mirrors of the mind. *Sci. Am.* 295 (5): 54–61.

Rizzolatti G., and L. Craighero. 2004. *The mirror neuron system. Ann Rev Neurosci* 27: 169–192.

———, and D. Sinigaglia. 2006. *So quel che fai. Il cervello che agisce e i neuroni specchio.* Milano: Raffaello Cortina Editore.

———. 2007. Mirror neurons and motor intentionality. *Funct. Neurol.* 22 (4): 205–10.

———. 2008. Further reflections on how we interpret the action of others. *Nature* 2, 455 (7213): 589.

———. 2010. The functional role of the parieto-frontal mirror circuit: interpretations and misinterpretations. *Nat. Rev. Neurosci.* 11 (4): 264–74.

Rizzolatti, G., and L. Vozza. 2008. *Nella mente degli altri. Neuroni specchio e comportamento sociale.* Bologna: Zanichelli.

———. 2005. The mirror neuron system and its function in humans. *Anat. Embryol.* 210 (5–6): 419–21.

Rockland, K.S., and D.N. Pandya. 1979. Laminar Origins and Terminations of Cortical Connections of the Occipital Lobe in the Rhesus Monkey. *Brain Research,* 179: 3–20.

Rosanova, M. 2012. Recovery of cortical effective connectivity and recovery of consciousness in vegetative patients. *Brain.* 135 (Pt 4): 1308–20.

Royal College of Physicians of London. 2003. The vegetative state: guidance on diagnosis and management. *Clin Med* 3: 249–254.

Sabatano, C. 2003, *Dal corpo alla mente. Prospettive teoriche e metodologie formative,* Napoli: Liguori.

———. 2004. *Come si forma la memoria. Ipotesi sperimentali di ricerca bioeducativa.* Roma: Carocci.

———. 2005. *Formare al senso di sé. Percorsi e problemi pedagogici.* Pisa: Edizioni ETS.

Sakai, K., and Y. Miyashita. 1991. Neural organization for the long-term potentiation memory of paired associates. *Nature* 354: 152–155.

Salmeri, G. 2013. *Determinazioni dell'affetto.* Roma: Aracne.

Salomon, G. (ed.). 1993. *Distributed Cognitions. Psychological and Educational Considerations.* Cambridge: Cambridge University Press.

Santerini, M. 2011. *Educazione morale e neuroscienze. La coscienza dell'empatia*. Brescia: La Scuola.

Santoianni, F., M. Striano, and F. Frauenfelder. 2000. *Immagini e teorie della mente*. Roma: Carocci Editore.

———. 2003, *Modelli teorici e metodologici dell'apprendimento*. Roma-Bari: Editrice Laterza.

Santoianni, F., and C. Sabatano. 2002. *Architetture cognitive. Apprendimenti e memorie*. Lecce: Pensa Multimedia.

———. 1998. *Sistemi biodinamici e scelte formative*. Napoli: Liguori.

———. 2003. *Sviluppo e formazione delle strutture della conoscenza. Tendenze di ricerca nella pedagogia contemporanea*. Pisa: Edizioni ETS,

———. 2006. *Educabilità cognitiva. Apprendere al singolare, insegnare al plurale*. Roma: Carocci.

———. 2012. *L'approccio bioeducativo alla letto-scrittura*. Gardolo (Tn): Centro Studi Erickson.

Sbattella, L. 2006. *La mente orchestra. Elaborazione della risonanza e autismo*. Milano: Vita e Pensiero.

Schacter, D.L. 2001a. *The seven sins of memory: How the mind forgets and remembers*. Boston: Houghton Mifflin.

———. 2001b. *Forgotten ideas, neglected pioners: Richard Semon and the story of memory*. Philadelphia: Psychology Press.

Schiff, N.D. 2006. Multimodal neuroimaging approaches to disorders of consciousness. *J. Head Trauma Rehabil.* 21: 388–397.

Schwartz, J.H. 1971. Functioning of identified neurons and synapses in abdominal ganglion of Aplysia in absence of protein synthesis. *Journal of Neurophysiology* 34: 939–953.

Searle, J. 1983. *Intentionality: an essay in the philosophy of mind.* New York: Cambridge University Press.

———. 1984. *Minds, Brains and science.* Cambridge (MA): Harvard University Press.

———. 1992. *The rediscovery of the mind.* Cambridge, London: MIT Press.

———. 1997. *The Mystery of Consciousness*. New York: The New York Review of Books.304

———. 2001. *Rationality in Action*. Cambridge: The MIT Press.

———. 2002. *Consciousness and language.* Cambridge: Cambridge

University Press.

———. 2004. *Mind. A Brief Introduction.* Oxford: Oxford University Press.

———. 2007. *Freedom and Neurobiology: Reflections on free will, language, and political power*. New York: Columbia University Press

———. 2008. *Philosophy in a New Century: Selected Essays*. Cambridge: Cambridge University Press.

———. 2010. *Making the social world: the structure of human civilization.* Oxford: Oxford University Press.

Semplici, S. 2009a. Il disincanto e la stranezza fino a un certo punto. In *Natura in etica*, eds, F. Botturi and R. Mordacci. Milano: Vita e Pensiero, 3–24.

———. 2009b. Il vissuto della mente e la sfida della neuroetica. *Idee* 70: 153–67.

Serulle, Y. et al. 2007. A novel GluR1-cGKII interaction regulates AMPA receptor trafficking. *Neuron* 56: 670–688.

Shannon C.E 1948. The mathematical theory of communication, *B.S.T. Jour*. 27:379–423; 623–656

———, Weaver W. 1949. *The Mathematical Theory of Communication.* Urbana (IL): University of Illinois Press.

Shaw, R. 1981. Strange Attractors, Chaotic Behavior, and Information Flow. *Z. Naturforsch* 36a: 80–112.

Siegel, D. J. 1995. Perception and cognition. In *Comprehensive Textbook of Psychiatry*, eds. B. Kaplan, and W. Sadock. Baltimore: Williams&Wilkins.

———. 1996. Dissiociation, psychotherapy and the cognitive sciences. In *The Treatment of Dissociative Identity Disorder*, ed. J. Spira. San Francisco: Jossey-Bass.

———. 1999. *The Developing Mind*. New York: Guilford Press.

———. 2001. Toward an interpersonal neurobiology of the developing mind: attachment, 'mindsight,' and neural integration. *Infant Mental Health Journal* 22:67–94.

———. 2003. An interpersonal neurobiology of psychotherapy: The developing mind and the resolution of trauma. In *Healing Trauma*, eds. M. Solomon, and D. J. Siegel. New York: W.W. Norton, 1–56.

———. 2006. An interpersonal neurobiology approach to psychotherapy. *Psychiatric Annals*, 36 (4): 248–256.

———. 2007. *The Mindful Brain: Reflection and attunement in the cultivation of well-being*. New York (NY): W W Norton & Co.

Sinigaglia, C. and G. Rizzolatti. 2011. Through the looking glass: self and others. *Conscious Cogn*. 20 (1): 64–74.

Squire, L.R., and S. Zola-Morgan. 1991. The medial temporal lobe memory system. *Science* 253: 1380–1386.

———, E.K. Kandel, and S.M. Kosslyn. 1996. Cognitive neuroscience. *Curr. Opin. Neuobiol*. 6 (2): 153–7.

———, and P.J. Bayley. 2007. The neuroscience of remote memory. *Current Opinion in Neurobiology* 17: 185–196.

———, and E.K. Kandel. 2009. *Memory: from mind to molecules*. Colorado: Roberts & Company.

———. 1987. *Memory and Brain*. New York: Oxford University Press.

———. 1989. On the course of forgetting in very long-term memory. *Journal of Experimental Psychology: Learning, Memory and Cognition* 15: 241–245.

———. 1992. Memory and the hippocampus: a synthesis from findings with rats, monkeys, and humans. *Psychol. Rev*. 99 (2): 195–231.

———. 2004. Memory systems of the brain: a brief history and current perspective. *Neurobiol. Learn. Mem*. 82 (3): 171–177.

———. 2007. Neuroscience. Rapid consolidation. *Science* 316 (5821): 57–58.

———. 2009. The legacy of patient H.M. for neuroscience. *Neuron* 61(1): 6–9.

Stein E. 1917. *Zum problem der Einfuehlung*. Halle: Buchdruckerei des Waisenhausen.

Stern, D. N. 1985. *The Interpersonal World of the Infant*. New York: Basic Books.

Sternberg, R. J., and E. Grigorenko. (eds.). 1997. *Intelligence, Heredity, and Environment*. New York: Cambridge University Press.

Steward, O. 1997. mRNA localization in neurons: A multipurpose mechanisms? *Neuron* 18: 9–12.

Strata, P., W.T. Thach, and O.P. Ottersen. 2009. New insights in cerebellar function. Introduction. *Neuroscience*. 162(3): 545–8.

Strollo M.R. 2008. *Laboratorio di ępistemologia e di pratiche dell'educazione. Un approccio neuro fenomenologico alla formazione pedagogica degli educatori*. Napoli: Liguori.

Tadié, J. Y. And M. Tadié. 1999. *Le sens de la mémoire*. Paris: Gallimard.

Tanzella-Nitti, G. 2009. *Faith, Reason and the Natural Sciences. The Challenge of the Natural Sciences in the Work of Theologians*. Aurora, CO: The Davies Group.

———. 2012a. Religion and science as inclinations toward the search for global meaning. *Theology and Science* 10 (2): 167–178.

———. 2012b. La questione antropologica in prospettiva teologica. In *Conversazioni su scienza e fede*, ed. Centro D.I.S.F. Torino: Lindau.

Tempia F, M. Bravin, and P. Strata. 1996. Postsynaptic currents and short-term synaptic plasticity in Purkinje cells grafted onto an uninjured adult cerebellar cortex. *Eur J Neurosci*. 8(12): 2690–701.

Thomas, A.K., and M.A. McDaniel. 2007. The negative cascade of incongruent generative study-test processing in memory and metacomprehension. *Memory and Cognition* 35: 668–678.

Thompson E. 2001. Empathy and Consciousness. In *Between Ourselves*, ed. E. Thompson. Thoverton: Imprinting Academic.

Tong, S., and N.V. Thakor. (eds.). 2009. *Quantitative EEG analysis methods and clinical applications*. Norwood (MA): Artech House.

Tonini V. 1983. *La scienza della vita*. Roma: Jouvence.

Tononi, G. 2004. An information integration theory of consciousness. *BMC Neurosci*. 5: 42.

———. 2012. Integrated information theory of consciousness: an updated account. *Arch.Ital. Biol.* 150 (4): 293–329.

———, and M. Massimini. 2013. A theoretically based index of consciousness independent of sensory processing and behavior. *Sci.Transl.Med*. 5(198): 198ra105.

Trevarthen, C. 1996. Lateral Asymmetries in Infancy: Implications for the Development of the Hemispheres. *Neuroscience and Biobehavioral Reviews* 20: 571–586.

Tulving, E. 1972. Episodic and semantic memory. In *Organization of memory*, eds. E. Tulving, and W. Donaldson. New York: Academic Press: 381–403.

———. 1995. Organisation of Memory: Quo Vadis? In *The Cognitive Neuroscience*, ed. M. S. Gazzaniga. Cambridge: MIT Press.

Turing, A.M. 1950. Computing machinery and intelligence, *Mind*, 59:433–460.

Varela, F. J., E. Thompson, and E. Rosch. 1991. *The Embodied Mind: Cognitive Science and Human Experience.* Cambridge: MIT Press.

———, and J. Shear. 1999. First person accounts: why, what and how. In *The view from within,* eds. F. J., Varela, and J. Shear. Bowling Green: Imprinting Academic.

———. 1979. *Principles of biological autonomy.* New York: Elsevier North Holland.

———. 1983. Self-organization: beyond appearances and into the mechanism, *La Nuova Critica* 64: 31–51.

———. 1990. Il corpo come macchina ontologica. Che Cos'è la conoscenza? In eds. M. Ceruti, and L. Preta. Roma: Laterza.

———. 1997. Patterns of life: intertwining identity and cognition. *Brain Cogn.* 34 (1): 72–87.

———. 1999. The specious present: a neurophenomenology of time consciousness. In *Naturalizing Phenomenology: Issues in Contemporary Phenomenology and Cognitive Science,* eds. J. Petitot, F.J. Varela, J.M. Roy and B. Pachoud. Stanford: Stanford University Press.

Vecchiato G. et al. 2009, The study of brain activity during the observation of commercial advertising by using high resolution EEG techniques. *Conf Proc IEEE Eng Med Biol Soc.*: 57–60.

Vitiello, G., and E. Pessa. 2003. Quantum Noise, Entanglement and Chaos in the Quantum Field Theory of Mind/Brain States. *Mind and Matter* 1 (1): 59–79.

———. 1997. Dissipazione e coscienza. *Atque* 16: 171–198.

———. 2003. Quantum dissipation and information. *NeuroQuantology* 1: 266–279.

———. 2004. The dissipative brain. In *Brain and Being,* eds. G. Globus, K. Pribram and G. Vitiello. Amsterdam and Philadelphia: John Benjamins.

———. 2009a. Io e il mio doppio: la dinamica coerente del cervello e l'emergenza della coscienza, *La Med. Biol.* 4: 9–15.

———. 2009b. Coherent states, fractals and brain waves. *New Mathematics and Natural Computing* 5: 245–264

Von Neumann, J. 1958. *The Computer and the Brain.* The New Haven: Yale University Press.

Waddington, C. H. 1957. *The Strategy of the Genes.* London: George

Allen and Unwin.

———. 1966. *Principles of Development and Differentiation*. New York: Macmillan.

Wang, H.G. et al. 2005. Presynaptic and postsynaptic roles of NO, cGK, and RhoA in long-lasting potentiation and aggregation of synaptic proteins. *Neuron*. 45(3): 389–403.

Warrington, E.K., and R. McCarthy. 1983. Category specific access dysphasia. *Brain* (Pt 4): 859–78.

Watson, J.B. 1930. *Behaviorism*. New York: W. W. Norton and Company.

Watson, J. and F. Crick. 1953. Molecular Structure of Nucleic Acids: A Structure for Deoxyribose Nucleic Acid. *Nature* 171: 737–738.

Weinberg, S. 1995. Reductionism redux. *New York Review of Books* 42: 39–42.

Wheeler, J.A. 1990. Information, physics, quantum: The search for links. In W. H. Zurek (ed.) *Complexity, entropy, and the physics of information*. Redwood City (CA): Addison-Wesley.

Wiener N. 1948. *Cybernetics or Control and Communication in the Animal and the Machine*. Cambridge, MA: MIT Press.

Wilson, E.O. 1980. *Sulla natura umana*. Bologna: Zanichelli.

Zeki, S. 1999. *Inner vision: an exploration of art and the brain*. London: Oxford University Press.

———. 2011. *Splendors and Miseries of the Brain examines the elegant and efficient machinery of the brain*. Oxford: John Wiley & Sons.

Zhang, Y. et al. 2011. Object decoding with attention in inferior temporal cortex. *Proc Natl Acad Sci U S A*.108(21): 8850–5.

Made in United States
Orlando, FL
04 November 2026

90206780R00157